THE RETURN OF THE ANCIENT SEED

HOW SALBA IS SHAPING MODERN NUTRITION

SHERRILL SELLMAN, N.D.

FOREWORD BY VLADIMIR VUKSAN, PH.D.

Author: Sherril Sellman
Editorial Director: Brian Keyes
Composition: Cory Goodspeed and Brian Keyes

Published 2008
All rights reserved

Published by
THC, INC. PUB
165 N. 100 E. Ste.2
St. George, Utah 84770

Copyright© 2008 Sherrill Sellman

ISBN 978-0-9793979-3-6

Printed in the United Sates of America

14 13 12 11 10 09 08   1 2 3 4 5

This book is available at quantity discounts for bulk purchases.
For information, please call: 1-888-499-8665.

CONTENTS

FOREWORD
BY VLADIMIR VUKSAN, PH. D.

I BEGAN PIONEERING the development of functional foods in Europe as part of an alternative and complementary treatment for chronic disease. My greatest interest was in the area of prevention of type 2 diabetes and reduction of heart disease risk factors, a great challenge that perseveres with me to this day. I was deeply motivated to investigate therapies or ingredients that could come closer to meeting the challenges of modern disease processes and still be natural, efficacious and safe. We soon realized that available treatments in the West do not yet provide the complete remedy, so we began to scour the world, looking for "old medicine" to treat modern diseases that could be combined with available treatments. Our investigations led us to many places - it gave us the fiber root from Japan; ginseng from Canada and the Orient; and most recently a phenomenal whole grain called Salba, which has been used for centuries in Central America.

Before I say more about Salba, I would like to elaborate on how we have approached the research and what we have discovered.In the last 20 years of working at the University of Toronto, I have tried intensively to expand our understanding of nutritional interventions, not only by investigating their capacity to prevent chronic disease, but also by developing functional foods that are able to actively treat or manage poor health such as type 2 diabetes and heart disease.

Over a period of 30 years, we have developed novel therapies that are able to improve important risk factors for heart disease. The therapies are based on highly viscous dietary fibers and medicinal plants, administered either alone or in combination. These therapies have proven to be quite effective in reducing conventional risk factors such as blood pressure and cholesterol and regulation of diabetes. However, these are only some of the problems associated with atherosclerotic changes in chronic diseases like type 2 diabetes and heart disease. These diseases encompass a cluster of conventional as well as novel risk factors that determine health complications and premature death risk. For other factors linked to the thrombotic aspects of type 2 diabetes, the so called novel risk factors, such as low-grade body inflammation and fibrinolysis (coagulation of the blood), there is currently no panacea even with conventional medicine.

Approximately 7 years ago, we were fortunate to begin extensive research on Salba, a new, intriguing and novel whole grain that interested me for at least two reasons. First, I was impressed with its long history of use as a food and remedy by the ancient Aztecs, an extraordinarily advanced civilization. And second, because of its superior nutrient composition which suggested potential health benefits even greater than many other foods and supplements that we had previously studied in our laboratory.

We were very eager to demonstrate Salba's health properties, and began a series of acute, and long-term studies in healthy individuals and those with well-controlled type 2 diabetes. The addition of Salba to their daily diet, combined with conventional medical treatment, had the ability to further improve metabolic control by lowering blood pressure, affecting low-grade body inflammation, and reducing blood clotting.

These preliminary findings were somewhat unexpected and remarkable – the magnitude of these clinical results is rarely seen with modern therapies. Data on this important study was published in the November 2007 issue of *Diabetes Care*, which is one of the leading and most prestigious diabetes journals in the world. It is also an official journal of the American Diabetes Association, which incidentally, rarely publishes nutritional studies.

Some of the data from the long term study conducted in our center was reproduced in a Belgian study at the University of Antwerp. These investigators found that the addition of Salba for four weeks to a regular diet in healthy individuals, improved their blood pressure, reduced their waist circumference, and decreased triglyceride levels. As we were unable to pinpoint a single factor of Salba that could cause such an effect, we have concluded that Salba, as a true functional food, is effective because it is a rich source of phytochemicals, including fiber, omega-3, minerals and antioxidants that have multiple interactions and act synergistically to produce desired health effects. After these very encouraging preliminary results we continued to study Salba with even more intensity and enthusiasm.

As we delved further into the explanation for some of the unexpected results, we decided to then investigate the role of Salba in glycemic control. The most recent dose-response acute study measured how Salba affects the after-meal blood glucose rise following white bread consumption, which is typically considered unhealthy due its high glucose raising characteristics. It was found that the addition of Salba to white bread produced a pronounced blood sugar lowering effect of approximately 30% compared to placebo, an effect that is considerably greater in comparison to that of other whole grains. The general conclusion from this project was that each gram of Salba added to white bread lowered blood sugar levels by 2% in healthy individuals. This means that, for example, the addition of only 1 tablespoon (12g) of Salba to white bread would result in a 24% reduction in blood glucose levels.

The other interesting finding was that the Salba enriched bread was able to significantly decrease appetite by on average more than 30% .This may have been partially due to having lower blood sugar levels after eating conventional white bread containing Salba. These results provide a preliminary platform and evidence for future research on Salba in battling obesity.

A further advantage of Salba is its simplicity of use which makes our studies easier to conduct and also allows consumers to incorporate Salba into almost any type of food or beverage. Adding Salba to any diet, good or bad, will improve its health profile and contribute to an individual's overall well-being. Its neutral flavor does not alter the taste of any food. This has prompted me to dub Salba a "Stealth Health" grain as its neutral flavor blends extremely well with any other ingredients.

Another important advantage to other grains or seeds is that Salba can be consumed either in its whole form or ground, with comparable health effects such as glucose lowering benefits,. Even where severe processing is involved, there will be no deleterious effect on the efficacy of the grain or any major impact on its nutrient composition.

Salba's encouraging clinical data is welcome news for people who wish to follow government recommendations to increase their whole grain consumption. New information appears almost daily on the important role that whole-grains play in the prevention of diabetes and heart disease. As most of the grains and cereal foods eaten today are refined and overly-processed, adding Salba to a daily diet may remedy this deficiency.

Salba can therefore be considered an excellent functional food, not only for its practicality, but also in its ability to address major public health problems that are related to our modern diet (empty calories and highly refined food) in developed societies as well as under-nutrition, a burden of developing countries.

We feel there is a great future for many applications of Salba due to its unique nutritional composition and preliminary clinical data. Based on the nutrient composition, it seems that Salba may be beneficial in every stage of life, particularly in children, women and the elderly, to preserve health and perhaps manage disease.

Although the data we have so far is very encouraging, more work needs to be done and our research team is eager to uncover further health benefits of this fascinating grain, especially in areas where Salba may have the most potential to create new health applications. Future studies will focus on possible ways that Salba can improve regularity and colon health, due to its potentially strong prebiotic effect, improve circulation and arterial stiffness and perhaps, as Salba's biggest challenge, battle weight loss, with obesity being a major public health problem.

Our team at the University of Toronto are convinced that because of its unique properties, Salba will be recognized and recommended by scientists, agronomists, government regulators, health agencies and consumers world-wide, irrespective of age group, gender, health conditions, lifestyle, profession or ethnicity, whether they live in America, Europe, Africa or Asia.

Salba – a cornucopia for the 21st century – and a grain set apart.

THE SALBA
JOURNEY

INTRODUCTION BY MITCH PROPSTER

IN THE SUMMER OF 2004 my occupation was buying and selling computer and technology equipment. And while I was making great money, my life lacked a certain fulfillment. In addition, health and nutrition were close to the bottom on my list of priorities. I can't recall the exact date, but I awoke one summer day and decided that selling technology was no longer my life's plan, and it was time for something better. More importantly, it was time for something that was going to give back to society.

A friend and roommate who lived a strict fitness regimen came to me and said, "Hey Mitch, why don't we start a nutrition supply company?" At that time I was using e-commerce technologies to sell my products and while the use of that technology was not a complete departure from my past, it would provide me a segue into what would become my future enterprise in so many more ways than I could have ever imagined.

My immediate thoughts were keeping a paycheck coming in, so in my style of risk taking, I agreed, and immediately began building what was known at that time as "NutriCell". This company would provide nutritional products in a user-friendly interface allowing the public to easily find health and wellness products for a variety of needs.

This initial version of the website carried over 300 items, many of them very well known at that time. Within months, I had established a pretty good business and a loyal customer following. Interestingly, I would get calls from time to time with praise for one product or another and I recall how nice it was to hear that people were actually receiving benefit from how I made my living. These calls drove me to want to learn more about what I believe now is the most incredible industry in our country.

Several more months passed by, and during the summer of 2005 a colleague called to tell me that I needed to fly to Atlanta right away. He was extremely excited about something new; introduced to him by some farmers in Peru. Curious, I was on a plane within a few days.

My friend was running a boutique manufacturing house from which I bought unique formulas to market. Naturally, I wanted to find out what this exciting new product was and with great anticipation, I waited as he brough it out...a foil bag full of small, plain, white seeds.

Needless to say, I was not awestruck. I was expecting something far more exciting or cutting-edge than a bunch of tiny seeds in a bag.

Perplexed, I asked "What's so good about these?" He immediately broke into a riveting and multi-faceted explanation that included EFA's, fiber, minerals, and amino acids. I replied "All that's in these tiny seeds? What's it called?" He said "Salba".

I had so many more questions than could be answered at that time, so placing trust in my friend, I decided to test Salba's appeal on my web site. My staff and I worked diligently to educate people about the value of this new product, which prompted ongoing research on our part. After several calls to my friend, he finally directed me to a person with the answers: Larry Brown.

Larry worked alongside the farmers that grew Salba, and was instrumental in providing the wealth of information I needed to educate our customers. In October of 2005, I sold the first bottle of Salba. These unique seeds were so scarce at the time; they fetched $40.00 per pound, but the amazing thing was the frequency of incoming referrals and reorders for Salba. I had never witnessed anything like it.

As I wondered to myself what was so great about this seed called Salba, I got a call that literally changed the way I viewed both the product, and this industry. It was this profound call that fueled my motivation for my new way of life, and it was everything I needed.

The call was from an elderly woman in her mid- to late-eighties. I could feel her energy coming through the receiver. She asked, "May I speak to the person responsible for allowing me to have this wonderful product?" I said, "Well ma'am, that would be the farmers but they are in Peru, so I guess I will have to do!" She went on to tell me that she and her husband were recovering cancer patients, and the chemo-therapy they had received had all but drained them of their daily energy. So much so she told me that all they could do was sit, or lay around the house with very little or no activity.

She went on to say that a friend had recently called her to rave about Salba, and that she started taking it approximately 15 days prior to this call. She literally began to cry and told me that as a result of consuming Salba both she and her husband were able to perform chores around the house and lead somewhat normal lives – she said "you have given us 10 years of our lives back, and we want to thank you!"

Never had I heard such a thing first hand and I was beside myself with emotion. At that moment I realized the power of Salba and that I could have a hand in helping more people to feel this well and that really excited me. More and more calls of the same nature began to pour in, and then letters and emails – it was nothing short of spectacular.

During the next few months Salba enjoyed growing popularity and as interest grew in the product, so did my interest in the natural products industry. I began attending expos and seminars and meeting some truly magnificent people whose main interest was in giving consumers natural and safe alternatives to western philosophies.

Larry called me one day and asked if I would be interested in representing Salba in the U.S. marketplace. I really did not know how to respond, but I knew if I was going to make a massive impact, I would need the right kind of fuel to make it a reality. Both Salba and the consumer provided the answer, so I agreed to meet with the Salba farming team in Miami.

When I was set to meet the Mealla brothers, I really had no concrete idea how I was going to execute this distribution plan – I only knew I had to, and that under any circumstances, I had to make it work. So I arrived with incredible plans, spreadsheets, and packaging ideas and more enthusiasm than I could harness.

The younger of the brothers, Alfredo, was a charming, youthful individual. At near fifty he was running marathons and flying all over the world supporting their business of experimental crops. He explained to me the 15 year process of how they arrived at the unique seeds we know today as Salba. The development of the proprietary growing standards that earned them the only known registered variety of this botanical, the unique harvesting and irrigative conditions, the best known growing locations, the agronomic science of NON-GMO selective breeding, and most importantly, the research that would prove the efficacy of what they had been laboring over.

The story was overwhelming, but I still had one really important question to ask...why? Why would they take fifteen years, a considerable amount of money, all the time resource and energy and even some failures to arrive at today? So I inquired and the answer was so impactful in its simplicity... Alfredo told me, "If we can grow enough Salba, we can feed hungry nations." Honestly, I was not expecting this answer, and it really caught me off guard – I now had the final reason I needed...and in that meeting, my life and what I was going to do with it changed forever.

I aligned myself with this endeavor and decided the best way I could contribute was by building a market for this incredible little seed. Alfredo and I decided our first steps of action. These plans included the founding of Core Naturals, which would serve as the premier U.S distributor of Salba.

We sealed the deal with a handshake!

In early 2008, Salba by Core Naturals was the first whole food and functional ingredient to be recognized by NutraCon as one of the top three finalists for best new product in the industry among well over 1,500 submissions.

Today, Salba is sold in over 5,000 retail stores nationwide, offered through multiple channels of distribution, and distributed to over six countries other than the U.S. Salba enjoys continual growth with one of the highest compliance and retention rates of any natural product.

Many people ask me who my inspiration was and who fueled my passion for bringing Salba to the U.S.

While the story of the Mealla brothers farming team, contributors like Larry and Trudy Brown, and other Salba partners have shaped what Salba is today, there is no greater inspiration for me than you; the reader, our consumer – for it is for you that I have personally challenged myself to please on every level, and from every facet of the Core Naturals organization.

The health conscious consumer is the very reason for our existence, and we exist today because of your ongoing and valuable input, desire, and daily need for genuine health and wellness that can be delivered through this one-of-a-kind food we call Salba. And for that I am eternally grateful.

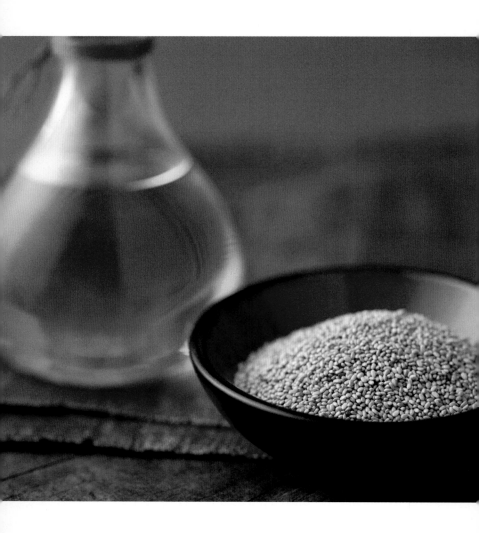

CHAPTER ONE

SEEKING A MIRACLE CURE?

SOMETHING UNUSUAL has been happening in Appleton, Wisconsin. To be more specific, some big changes have occurred at Central Alternative High School. As you walk through its halls, you will see students intently focused on their schoolwork, interacting peacefully with each other and their teachers. Students here are happy and eager to learn. But, this wasn't always the case.

The Appleton Central Alternative High School was established in 1996 for troubled kids barred from attending traditional high school because of discipline problems. Things were so bad at Appleton that a police officer was stationed full time at the school to prevent violence and weapons violations. Revolving discipline plans, metal detectors, security officers, and all the tactics used to deal with rowdy; violent teens were part of the typical school day.

What changed all this? Food! Wholesome, nutritious, real food. In 1997, a five-year project was initiated to bring healthy foods into the school program. Out went the soda and candy vending machines along with greasy burgers, fries and white bread. In came salads, wholesome meat recipes, fresh fruits and whole grain breads.

And then the miracles began to happen. The violent, unruly and inattentive kids transformed into exemplary students. Since incorporating a healthy, nutrient- rich diet for school lunches, no one has dropped out, no one has been expelled, no one has been found using drugs or carrying weapons and there have been no suicides. What's even more amazing, the students were thinking more clearly; they were healthier; they were more emotionally balanced; and they significantly improved their academic performance.

The lesson learned from the Appleton Central High School experience was profound. Nourish the body with nutritious, nutrient-dense food and a healthy happy and intelligent human being emerges!

We've Got Plenty of Nothing

WE LIVE IN A COUNTRY of plenty. Our plates are piled high with mounds of food. The supermarket shelves are fully stocked with rows and rows of canned, frozen, preserved and packaged foods. Restaurants and fast food chains, offer super-sized, jumbo, whopper meals. Food is everywhere.

However, there is a big difference between an abundance of food and an abundance of nutrition. We can feel full but still be malnourished.

Most Americans think of malnutrition only in its extreme as seen in pictures of skin and bone people wasting away and dying in impoverished countries. In reality, malnutrition is "a lack of necessary or proper food substances in the body or improper absorption and distribution of them."

Food that once came fresh from the farm is now created in top secret laboratories manned by teams of food scientists. Some of our favorite foods are a chemical potpourri without a trace of a natural ingredient to be found anywhere.

The average North American's daily menu consists of an over-consumption of empty calories, toxic fats, refined carbohydrates, excessive sugar, chemically infused meats, and artificial preservatives and flavorings. Our preferences for such foods are, in no stretch of the imagination, a recipe for good health!

Nutrition-related diseases are the leading American diseases today – heart disease, obesity, diabetes, colon cancer and most cancers, etc. Clinical deficiencies are also at the root of new illnesses unheard of before the 20th Century -- Chronic Fatigue, Fibromyalgia, Immune Dysfunction, PMS, Anxiety or Panic Attacks, Bi-Polar Disorder, ADD, ADHD, etc.

It is reported that 98.5 percent of the U.S. population are unhealthy. That only leaves 1.5 percent of us as fighting fit specimens.

How did this happen? Dr. Royal Lee, known as the father of nutritional medicine, answered this very question in 1943.

"We have drifted into this deplorable position of national malnutrition quite inadvertently. It's the result of scientific research to create foods that are non-perishable, mass-produced, and distributed so cheaply. Then, after a suspicion develops that these foods are inadequate to support life, modern science and advertisers then step in to get people to believe there is nothing wrong with them, so the confused public continues to blindly buy the rubbish that is killing them off years ahead of their time."

The legacy of our modern Western Diet is the declining health of our children. Today, our children are being born with more mental and physical health challenges and developing adult-type diseases in their youth.

Before our very eyes, American children (as well as children around the world) are becoming obese. Since 1960, the incidence of childhood obesity has increased fifty percent, and about one fifth of American youngsters weigh more than they should.

The U.S.D.A. has reported that only 36.4 percent of U.S. children between the ages of 2 and 19 eat the recommended three to five servings of vegetables per day, and only 26 percent eat the two to four recommended daily servings of fruit.

■ **17**

It is truly alarming to discover a survey found that for today's toddlers, french fries are the number one 'vegetable' consumed!

Salba - Looking Back to the Future

IT IS TIME, once again, to follow the wisdom of ancient healers. "Let your food be your medicine and your medicine your food" summed up one of the key principles espoused more than 2500 years ago in ancient Greece by Hippocrates, the father of medicine. His golden rule highlighted the importance of good nutrition as the foundation for optimal wellbeing. In ancient Greece, food was used to treat both physical and psychological illnesses, and a physician giving diet inadequate attention was reason enough for a malpractice suit.

Could the elixir of good health actually be found in bioavailable nutrition of nutrient-dense foods? These are foods, which are rich in the nutrients that are vital for the body's ability to nourish, create energy, repair, regenerate and detoxify. Nutrient dense foods are abundant in vitamins, minerals, fiber, antioxidants, essential fatty acids and proteins.

Our modern world is truly in desperate need of nutrient dense, super-hero foods! One such super-hero food that has recently come to our rescue is a tiny power-packed seed from South America called Salba. This ancient seed was a primary source of nutrition highly valued by the great Aztec Empire.

With the help of modern science, the nutritional secrets of Salba are being revealed. These amazing discoveries are sending a wave of excitement throughout the nutritional world.

Throughout the pages of this book, you will learn about the extraordinary health benefits bestowed upon us from this ancient seed. You will also discover why Salba is considered nature's perfect whole food.

CHAPTER TWO

THE ANCIENT
SUPER
SEED

SALBA IS A VERY ANCIENT FOOD. The original variety of this seed was known by its botanical name, *Salvia Hispanica L.* It is believed the origins of Salba extended back thousands of years. In fact, evidence indicates that this species was an important food crop as early as 3500 BC. It also served as a cash crop in central Mexico between 1500 and 900 BC. A member of the mint family and also known by the ancients as chian, this seed played an especially important role in the culture of the Aztec Empire.

A powerful new civilization emerged in Mexico in the early 1400's who called themselves the Aztecs. This brilliant civilization controlled a region stretching from the Valley of Mexico in central Mexico, east to the Gulf of Mexico and south to Guatemala.

The Aztecs were renowned for their outstanding accomplishments in architecture, agriculture, horticulture and healing. The people of this incredible culture were refined workers, merchants, farmers and fishermen. They were also fierce warriors who possessed great stamina and strength.

Their stable crops included corn, beans and amaranth. However, there was another important staple food that was especially honored for its ability to create the powerful Aztec culture. That food was the seed then known as *chian* (oily seed).

The Aztecs believed it bestowed mystical, almost supernatural energy and power. It was so highly valued as a source of energy, endurance, strength and good health that the seeds were received as tribute from conquered nations and were given as offerings during religious ceremonies. This seed even became legal tender throughout the empire.

The Aztecs consumed these seeds in a variety of ways. They were eaten alone, mixed with other seed crops, made into a beverage, ground into flour, included in medicines, and pressed for oil.

According to Spanish manuscripts, the Aztecs consumed the seeds to sustain them on long and arduous hunting and trading expeditions. They called it their "running food" because messengers reportedly could run all day on just a handful of these nutrient-packed seeds.

The Aztec Empire met its demise with the arrival of the conquistador, Hernado Cortez in 1519. Cortez had an ambitious plan - to conquer the Aztec people and all their lands for the glory of Spain and, of course, himself! With a small army and the assistance of disaffected Indian tribes subjected by the Aztecs, Cortez successfully attacked and ultimately destroyed the Aztec Empire. By 1521, Cortez quickly realized that the crop was at the very core of the Aztec nutritional foundation. He was convinced that if he could destroy this source of sustenance, it would contribute to his defeat of the Aztecs.

The ruthless Conquistadors proceeded to burn the fields that grew this life-giving seed. In the end, the complete destruction of this food contributed to the triumph of Cortez and the end of the glorious Aztec Empire.

All knowledge of this amazing seed became lost in the midst of time after the conquistadors destroyed its cultivation. It is known that the Conquistadors brought some of the *Salvia* seeds back to Spain. Unfortunately, because the growing conditions were not appropriate for its successful cultivation, the crop was abandoned. Its glory days were eventually forgotten and the plant was relegated by the Spanish as a useless weed.

The famed botanist Carl Linnaeus who lived in the 1700's gave this seed its botanical name *Salvia hispanica L*, (the Latin word for Spain is Hispanica) which by this time had been growing wild in Spain and was mistakenly classified as a species native to that country. For more than 500 years, all knowledge of this nutritional powerhouse was all but forgotten.

Emerging from the Midst of Time

LIKE SO MANY SECRETS from ancient times, the nutritional legacy of this amazing seed would have remained forgotten if it weren't for the courage and vision of two Argentinean brothers.

Adolfo and Alfredo Mealla are successful South American farmers. Their family has farmed in South America for several generations. As innovative farmers, they are always on the lookout for new and beneficial crops.

In 1991, they were introduced to the original *Salvia* species. Preliminary tests showed this seed contained impressive amounts of omega-3 fatty acids. However, there were some problems with the earliest generations, which made it unsuitable for commercial agriculture. First, and most importantly, it did not have consistent essential fatty acid content. Some crops would yield as little as 15 percent omega-3's while others would have as much as 35 percent. In order to have a new food accepted into the market, nutritional consistency is imperative. This consistency was sorely lacking in the native varieties.

Another stumbling block was

the color, which were mostly black mixed with some white seeds. Black seeds would be visually difficult to incorporate into commercial products and ultimately hinder its mass appeal in the marketplace. It was believed not many people would really enjoy eating blackish/grayish colored cereals or muffins!

If this experimental crop was to succeed, it must have a consistent and stable essential fatty acid and overall nutritional profile as well as a color that could be an acceptable ingredient for a variety of products.

The Mealla brothers decided to gamble on this new crop by investing a great deal of their time and energy and, of course, financial resources, into traditional plant breeding techniques. Their goal was to create a white variety with a consistently high amount of omega-3 fatty acids and a stable overall nutrient density.

Their gamble ultimately paid off. After a decade of meticulous plant breeding to maximize its nutritional benefits, they successfully cultivated two-registered Non-GMO, varieties of white seeds known as, Sahi Alba 911 and Sahi Alba 912.

The name Salba was created by combining the letters of these two registered varieties.

Ancient Seed – Modern Sustainable Farming Practices

SALBA IS NOW GROWN exclusively in the mineral rich soils of an ideal climate in coastal Peru. (Salba thrives in a sunny, dry environment.)

Only the best sustainable agriculture practices are used. No chemicals or pesticides are used in any stage of its cultivation. Salba is allowed to fully ripen naturally in the field before being harvested. After harvest, all debris is eliminated from the seed, and then packaged into 25 kg. bags. It is then shipped to North America where it is stored in a climate-controlled environment.

The Mealla's had hoped their plant breeding efforts would pay off with an omega-3 rich seed that was commercially viable. But what has since been discovered about Salba has certainly surpassed their wildest expectations.

Salba is unlike any other variety of *Salvia hispanica L* found anywhere in the world. After more than a decade of testing, no single food is known to match Salba's nutritive power. Research has discovered that Salba contains an impressive amount of health-promoting omega-3 fatty acids, and is unusually high in dietary fiber.

In fact, Saba is the richest whole food source of omega-3 fatty acids and fiber in the world.

But there was more good news. In addition to its omega-3 content, it has also been discovered this tiny seed holds a whole world of nutrition within. It has complete, usable proteins; it is extremely rich in minerals such as calcium, magnesium, iron, and potassium; it contains high amounts of Vitamin C and other vitamins; and it is rich in vital age-fighting antioxidants.

The Mealla brothers are proud of their accomplishment in successfully breeding a new variety of this ancient seed. However, they take the greatest pride in knowing their painstaking efforts to develop Salba will help to nourish people desperately in need of nutrient-dense, functional food.

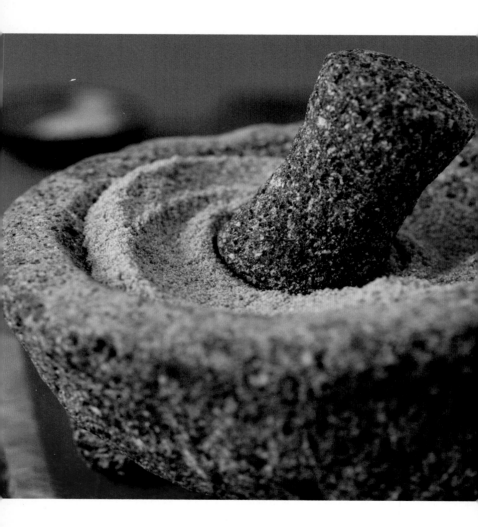

CHAPTER THREE

THE ULTIMATE FUNCTIONAL FOOD

THERE IS A NEW TERM in the lexicon of nutrition. It is called "functional foods". This category of foods refers specifically to those foods that have exceptional health benefits and disease preventing properties. From a therapeutic perspective, functional foods contain high amounts of powerful nutrients that have been proven to sustain and repair the body. They go far above and beyond the line of duty when it comes to providing the basic nutritional requirements for our daily needs.

In addition to functional foods, there is another important food type that also has a profound impact on your health. Known as nutrient-dense foods, these are foods that are particularly abundant in vitamins and minerals (micronutrients) but low in calories.

Nutrient-dense foods are opposite to the foods found in the average American diet i.e. energy-dense foods (also called "empty calorie" foods). According to *The Dietary Guidelines for Americans* (published jointly by the Department of Health and Human Services and the Department of Agriculture), fruits and vegetables are considered nutrient-dense foods, while products containing added sugars, saturated fats, and alcohol are considered nutrient-poor foods.

Functional foods and nutrient–dense foods play a vital role in ensuring you maintain optimal wellness at any age. They are particularly necessary to help you resolve any illness or chronic disease.

Hippocrates words ring true once more. "Leave your drugs in the chemist's pot if you can heal the patient with food." Thanks to the emergence of functional and nutrient-dense foods, we are, once again, learning how to heal by leaving behind the chemist's pot!

"Heal the patient with food" is a mantra well worth repeating in the 21st century.

Dynamic & Proven

ACCORDING TO DR. VLADIMIR VUKSAN, there is one exceptional functional food that stands out amongst all the rest. That super food is Salba.

Dr. Vuksan should know. He is one of the world's leading experts in the field of functional foods.

Dr. Vuksan's many accomplishments are quite impressive. He has held advisory and scientific positions with the prestigious World Health Organization and International Diabetes Federation. He is currently a Professor with the Department of Nutritional Sciences, Faculty of Medicine at the University of Toronto, and the Associate Director of the Clinical Nutrition and Risk Factor Modification Centre of St. Michael's Hospital in Toronto.

Dr. Vuksan's long career in the field of nutrition has established him as one of the most eminent authorities within the field of nutrition dedicated to developing novel alternative therapies for obesity, diabetes and heart disease.

He is also one of the world's leading researchers committed to unlocking the nutritional secrets hidden within Salba. Recent scientific studies have shown Salba to be nutritionally superior to many of today's popular health foods.

In fact, Dr. Vuksan emphatically states, "Salba can be considered a 'perfect' functional food."

How can Dr. Vuksan make such a bold claim?

Dr. Vuksan's research found that as a functional food, Salba achieved two world firsts. Its first claim to fame was it had the highest known whole food source of omega-3 fatty acids in the world. Omega-3 fatty acids are crucial for good health; regulating heart rate, blood pressure, blood clotting, fertility, immune support, improving mental health and reducing body inflammation. The National Institute of Health believes that most people need to at least double or triple their daily intake of Omega 3-Fatty Acids. This is where Salba comes to the rescue.

Just one tablespoon (12 grams) offers over 2.5 grams of omega-3 fatty acids (in an optimal 3 to 1 ratio), supplying more than 100 percent of the recommended daily intake.

If that wasn't impressive enough to make a superstar out of Salba, Dr. Vuksan also discovered Salba has the highest soluble and insoluble dietary fiber content of any grain currently on the market, providing more than four grams in just one tablespoon.

Fiber not only increases bulk and transit time and alleviates constipation, but also helps to maintain both healthy blood glucose and blood cholesterol levels. With such high fiber content, Salba provides superior ammunition in the battle of the bulge. Salba has the ability to absorb as much as 14 times its weight in water. When added to meals it becomes a bulking agent, ensuring slower digestion and a slower rise in blood sugar. Salba's fiber content, thus, stabilizes blood sugar levels, along with creating a sense of fullness.

Dr. Vuksan had even more good news on the nutrient-dense food front. When measuring nutrients gram for gram, Salba has six times more calcium than whole milk, three times more iron than spinach, the potassium content of 1 1/2 large bananas, fifteen times more magnesium than broccoli, and three times the antioxidant capacity of blueberries. In addition, Salba has much vitamin C as seven oranges.

Adding to this long list, Salba contains naturally occurring folate, B vitamins, zinc, selenium, and vitamin A. Salba also has more bioavailable and complete protein than rice, corn, oats, amaranth, soy, barley and wheat.

When it comes to antioxidants, Salba contains an arsenal of some of today's most potent age-fighting antioxidants, all in their natural form.

Overall antioxidant power of foods and supplements is measured by a test called ORAC, which stands for Oxygen Radical Absorbance Capacity. Since antioxidants are essential to good health, especially with respect to aging and age related disorders, the higher the ORAC value of a food the more antioxidant power it contains. The focus on "foods" is significant as scientists have found antioxidants are most effective when received from a whole food.

When measured on the ORAC test, Salba, whole seed, has a higher level of antioxidants than blackberries, strawberries, grapes, raisins, prunes, broccoli, cherries, and even spinach.

The really good news is even though Salba is such a high-powered food; it has less that 1/2 gm. net carbohydrate per serving.

And for all those people concerned about gluten foods, Salba is certified gluten-free as well as Non - GMO and kosher.

It's one thing finding a food that has superior nutrition, but it's another thing to have it acceptable to the American palate. That's where Salba also scores as a winner. Salba has a neutral flavor, which allows it to be an incredibly versatile food. Whether it is eaten as the whole seed, ground up as meal, or soaked in water and used as a gel, Salba can be a stealth ingredient fortifying an infinite variety of foods.

Dr. Vuksan has stated this about Salba: "Due to Salba's extremely high content of omega-3 fatty acids, and its nutrient-rich composition, Salba creates exceptional possibilities for the improvement of human health and nutrition. We continue to conduct studies on the vast benefits of this powerful grain and expect more promising results on the importance of adding Salba to our daily diet. Salba can be considered a perfect functional food."

IS SALBA THE "PERFECT" FUNCTIONAL FOOD?

Salba is a dynamic whole grain with a complete balance of vital nutrients, vitamins, and minerals - it blows other "super foods" out of the water.

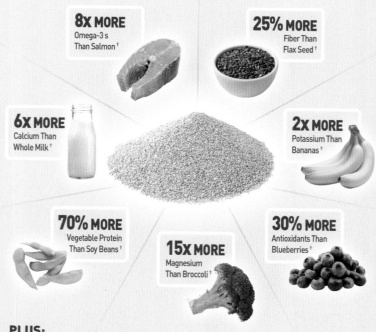

8X MORE
Omega-3 s
Than Salmon [†]

25% MORE
Fiber Than
Flax Seed [†]

6X MORE
Calcium Than
Whole Milk [†]

2X MORE
Potassium Than
Bananas [†]

70% MORE
Vegetable Protein
Than Soy Beans [†]

15X MORE
Magnesium
Than Broccoli [†]

30% MORE
Antioxidants Than
Blueberries [†]

PLUS:

6x More Iron Than Kidney Beans
15% More Fiber Than All Bran

5x More Iron Than Spinach
4x More Protein Than Kidney Beans

[†]Based on a gram-for-gram comparison using USDA nutritional data.

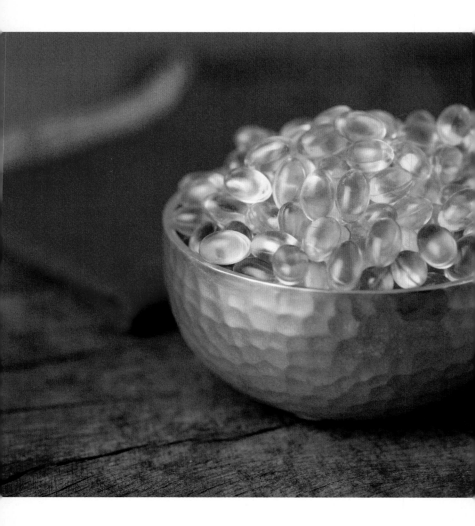

CHAPTER FOUR

THE ESSENTIAL
FATTY ACID
CHAMPION

HERE'S AN IMPORTANT QUESTION to ponder. When it comes to our health are fats the good guys or bad guys?

It certainly seems we live in a very fat phobic culture. Never before have Americans had so many low-fat, reduced-fat and fat-free foods to choose from. People avoid full fat versions like the plague! It seems to be a foregone conclusion that reducing fats or, even better, eliminating fats from the diet is a good health decision. But, do you really want a skinny latte with that fat-free muffin and fat-reduced cream cheese?

The perceived virtues of a "fat-free" world have profoundly influenced our thinking about fats as well as altered our eating habits and food choices. The media seems to fan the flame of an anti-fat world by quoting admonitions from various "health experts."

But before we reach for another fat- reduced potato chip, it's time to get fat savvy.

First of all, fat is one of the three essential macronutrients, along with vitamins and minerals. At all stages of our life, our bodies absolutely require them to maintain tiptop health.

Here's the second really important point; we need to make some important distinctions when we talk about fats. Some fats are absolutely required for good health while other kinds of fats will actually contribute to chronic illness.

"All fats are not created equally," says Dr. Udo Erasmus, author of the book, "Fats That Heal, Fats That Kill." "Eating the 'Good Fats' will slim you, improve your circulation, and boost your energy. But eating the 'Bad Fats', even though you may lose weight, can lead to serious health problems - even heart attacks and cancer."

As a leading expert on fats and oils, Dr. Erasmus says diets rich in fat can improve your health, but only if they are the right fats. He emphasizes that people must learn that there are two types of fats: "good fats" and "bad fats."

The ABCs of the Good Fats

THE MAIN COMPONENT of all fats is called fatty acids which include saturated, monounsaturated or polyunsaturated. Fatty acids are found in oils and other fats that make up different foods. Fats containing a high proportion of saturated fatty acids are solid at room temperature. These are commonly known as saturated fats and are usually derived from animal sources e.g. butter, lard, and suet.

Most plant fats are high in either polyunsaturated or monounsaturated fats (except palm and coconut fat which are highly saturated). They will be liquid at room temperature.

Saturated and monounsaturated fats can be made in the human body from the food we eat. They do not necessarily need to be supplemented from our diet.

However, there are two different categories - or "families" of polyun-saturated fatty acids (PUFAs) that cannot be manufactured by the body. They are known as omega- 3 (alpha-linolenic acid) and omega-6 (linoleic acid). Omega-3 fatty acids are contained in some plant oils and fish while omega-6 fatty acids are contained only in plant oil.

Omega-3 and omega-6 fatty acids are known as essential fatty acids. They are called "essential" because though they are critical for optimal health, they cannot be synthesized by the body. Since the body can not manufacture them, they must be obtained from the foods we eat.

The omega-3s are further converted into two other important forms of polyunsaturated fatty acids called EPA (eicosapentaenoic acid) and DHA (docosahexaenoic acid).

So, why are essential fatty acids such super nutritional stars? The following is an impressive list of the many important contributions EFAs have to your health.

Omega- 3s - Missing in Action

WHEN IT COMES to good health, balance is everything. This is especially true for essential fatty acids. The levels of essential fatty acids and the balance between them may play a critical role not only in growth and development, but also in the prevention and treatment of chronic diseases including coronary artery disease, hypertension, type II diabetes, arthritis and other immune/inflammatory disorders, and cancer.

Changes in our food supply since the industrial revolution have jeopardized both the quantity and balance of these nutrients. Modern foods and eating habits have the balance of essential fatty acid way out of whack.

Our diet contains excessive amounts of Omega-6 fats. These are the variety of vegetable oils like corn, soy, safflower and canola Omega-6 oils are found in thousands of processed food items found on supermarket shelves, in restaurants (especially fast food restaurants) and, most often, in our home pantries and refrigerators.

It seems that omega-6 oils have taken over our world. In just 100 years Americans have gone from consuming one pound per year to an estimated 75 pounds annually. That's put a lot of omega-6 into our bodies. At the same time omega-3 levels are now down to 16 percent of what people were able to consume over that same time period.

This over-zealous reliance on omega-6 oils creates a serious problem (apart from the fact they create toxic free-radicals). The all-important balance between omega-6 and omega-3 oils is seriously askew.

The Great Omega-3 Deficiency

EXPERTS LOOKING at the dietary ratio of omega-6 to omega-3 fatty acids, suggest that in early human history the ratio was about 1:1. Currently most Americans eat a dietary ratio that falls between 20:1 and 50:1. A healthy diet should consist of roughly two - four times more omega-6 fatty acids than omega-3 fatty acids. For most of us this means greatly reducing the omega-6 fatty acids we consume while increasing our intake of omega-3 fatty acids.

Dr. Artemis Simopoulos, an expert in essential fatty acids, writes that since 1960 our intake of omega-6 had nearly doubled and mirrors the increase of some of diet based diseases. She concludes," it seems increasingly likely the glut of omega-6 fatty acids in our diet is contributing to our high rates of cancer, depression and diabetes.

In a recent study, scientists concluded, "...we are now eating 1/10th of the amount of omega-3 required for normal functioning. Alarmingly, 20 percent of the population has levels so low that they defy detection." *(Dolocek, Grandits, World Rev. Nutr Diet. 1991, 66: 205-216)*

Both the National Institute of Health and the World Health Organization agree most people are severely deficient in omega-3s.

Omega-3 deficiency is the most common essential nutrient deficiency in the diet of most western societies. In fact, about 95-99 percent of the population is actually omega-3 deficient. (The next most common deficiencies are magnesium at about 85 percent and vitamin B6 at about 80 percent of the population.)

An omega-3 deficiency is also the single, most widespread, most health-damaging physical cause of degenerative diseases in our time. While omega-3 fatty acids help reduce inflammation, most omega-6 fatty acids tend to promote inflammation.

A number of studies have found that omega-3s significantly lowers the risk of death from heart disease. Omega-3s may also reduce risk of stroke as well as reducing elevated blood pressure. Research supports the fact that omega-3s reduce inflammation, reduce blood clotting, and ensure proper dilation of your blood vessels. Such impressive health benefits have convinced researchers omega-3s play a major role is preventing and mitigating chronic diseases such as heart disease, cancer, and arthritis.

TALK ABOUT "ESSENTIAL"

So, why are essential fatty acids such nutritional stars? Here's an impressive list of the many important contributions EFAs have to your health.

WHAT THEY DO	HOW THEY DO IT
INCREASE ENERGY, PERFORMANCE, & STAMINA	EFAs enhance thermogenesis, help build muscle, prevent muscle break down, and speed recovery from fatigue.
STRENGTHEN THE IMMUNE SYSTEM	EFAs make hormone-like eicosanoids that regulate immune and inflammatory responses. Omega -3's have anti-inflammatory effects and can slow autoimmune damage.
IMPROVE BRAIN FUNCTION: MOOD, INTELLIGENCE, BEHAVIOR, & VISION	Our brain is over 60% fat. EFAs are important components of the entire nervous system. They are necessary to make the neurotransmitter serotonin. Depression and other brain diseases show decreased levels of Omega-3.
AID IN WEIGHT REDUCTION	EFAs help keep mood and energy up and suppress appetite, thereby aiding in weight loss. More recently, they have been found to block the genes that produce fat in the body (saturated and trans fat do not have this same effect) and increase thermogenesis.
REGULATE ORGANS & GLANDS	Liver and kidneys, adrenal and thyroid glands, and the production of male and female hormones need EFAs. They are needed for the production of prostaglandins, which regulate body functions such as blood clotting, blood pressure, fertility, heart rate as well as strengthening the immune system and reducing inflammation.
SPEED RECOVERY & HEALING	EFAs are necessary for cell growth and division. They form all cell membranes and regulate vital cell activity.
DECREASE INFECTION	EFAs have anti-fungal, anti-yeast, and anti-microbial properties, helping to protect against infections.
KEEP BONES STRONG	EFAs aid in the transport of minerals that keep bones and teeth strong, helping to prevent osteoporosis.
PROTECT GENETIC MATERIAL	EFAs regulate gene expression.
NOURISH SKIN, HAIR, & NAILS	Some of the first signs of EFA deficiency are dry, flaky skin, dull hair, and brittle nails.
STRENGTHEN THE BONES	EFAs improve mineralization of the bones together with calcium, Vitamin C, D, K, boron and many other building blocks of the skeleton.
IMPROVE UPTAKE OF NUTRIENTS	EFAs are required for absorption and storage of the fat-soluble vitamins, such as vitamins D, E, K and E.

Even the American Heart Association agrees that omega-3s have an impressive positive effect on our health. Large-scale epidemiologic studies suggest that people at risk for coronary heart disease benefit from consuming omega-3s from plants and marine sources.

Omega-3 fatty acids are necessary for cardiovascular health for the following reasons:

* **Supports a healthy cardiovascular system**

* **Maintains healthy cholesterol levels**

* **Decreases risk of arrhythmias, which can lead to sudden cardiac death**

* **Decreases triglyceride levels**

* **Decreases growth rate of atherosclerotic plaque**

* **Helps to lower blood pressure**

It is now evident the health and wellbeing of every member of the family will benefit from regularly eating omega-3 rich foods. Since there is limited storage of omega-3 fatty acids in our bodies, these fatty acids must be a regular part of the diet.

Salba, - Nature's Richest Whole Food Source of Omega-3s

IN THE LANGUAGE of the ancient Aztecs, the name of the original Salba seeds was *chian*, meaning oily seed. Modern scientific techniques have revealed that Salba is a good source of healthy essential fatty acids.

But what really astounded the scientists was the discovery Salba was the richest whole food source of omeg-3 fatty acids in the world. In fact, the oil content of the seed ranges between an impressive 29-33 percent.

Salba also possesses the highest combined percentage of alpha-linolenic and linoleic of any known food. And there was one more amazing discovery. Salba has the highest levels of alpha-linolenic acid known in any plant, an impressive 62-65 percent!

In a world, desperately in need of increasing dietary sources of omega-3s, Salba also contains the perfect balance of omega-3 to omega-6, in an ideal 4:1 ratio.

What does all this mean? Just one tablespoon (12 gm) provides about 2.7 gms. of Omega-3. That means you are getting more than 100 percent of the recommended daily intake!

Salba and Cardiovascular Health

IT IS NOW ACCEPTED medical wisdom that diet plays a major role in the prevention as well as the treatment of chronic disease. This is particularly true in regards to the epidemic of cardiovascular disease (CVD). Heart disease and strokes are the leading cause of death in the United States. CVD is no longer thought of as a disease that primarily affects men as they age. It is a killer of people in the prime of life, with more than half of all deaths occurring among women.

In searching for solutions, a great deal of interest has been directed towards the heart-healthy effects of omega-3 fatty acids. Sufficient levels of this essential fatty acid have the ability to lower triglycerides, blood pressure and reduce cardiovascular disease mortality.

One important study, called The Lyon Diet Heart Study (LDHS), investigated the cardio-protective effects of plant-based omega-3s. They were particularly interested to discover if omega-3s could help prevent a recurrence of heart attacks. The diet used in this study was high in alpha-linolenic acid.

All the participants achieved amazing results. There was a 70 percent reduction in mortality– more than double the other trials that had used omega-3s from fish. There was also a significant reduction in coronary 'events' and these protective effects were found to start quickly. Four years on, patients were still following the diet and their hearts were still being protected, and subsequent studies have confirmed the power of plant omega-3 fatty acids in protecting the heart.

This study produced profound findings. Not only was there conclusive evidence that omega-3 fatty acids were, indeed, cardio-protective for high-risk patients but that plant based omega-3s in the form of alpha-linolenic acid were even more protective than fish oils. The study also demonstrated that plant oils reduce the risk of dying from secondary heart attack by more than double that of fish oils; plant oils reduce the number of painful, non-fatal heart attacks; and there are long-term survival benefits from consuming plant oils.

Salba Protects against Cardiovascular Risks from Diabetes

THE FIRST LONG-TERM STUDY investigating Salba's health effects was recently published in the prestigious

Diabetes Care (Vol.30, No. 11). The impressive results proving that Salba lowers cardiovascular disease has catapulted this humble seed into center stage.

Dr. Vladimir Vuksan has been intrigued about the possible nutritional contributions of Salba in improving a variety of chronic illnesses. He and his multidisciplinary team at the Clinical Nutrition and Risk Factor Modification Centre at St. Michael's Hospital in Toronto conducted a clinical trial with 20 type 2 diabetes patients who consumed four tablespoons of Salba every day for three months.

It is known that people with diabetes are at an increased risk for heart attacks or strokes. Compared to people without diabetes, the risk of heart attacks is 1.5 to 4.5 times greater for women and 1.5 to 2 times greater for men. Also, the risk of stroke is 2 to 6.5 times greater among women with type 2 diabetes and 1.5 to 2 times greater for men. Therefore, it is of utmost importance to find new functional foods for the treatment of diabetes.

Could Salba act as a functional food offering proven cardio-protective benefits in diabetic patients?

During the trial, the following results were observed:

* **Salba reduced after-meal blood glucose and plasma insulin levels, thus improving the Glycemic Index of any food consumed with Salba.**

* **C-reactive protein, a marker for low grade body inflammation was significantly lowered (40 percent).**

* **Salba reduced blood pressure, lowering systolic blood pressure, on average, by six points mmHg (millimeters of mercury).**

* **Salba significantly decreased coagulation (blood thinning) by 30 percent.**

* **No adverse effect was noted on glycemic control or blood lipids as previously seen with high doses of omega-3 fatty acids.**

The study also discovered that eating Salba increased levels of EPA (eicosapentaenoic acid), the particular kind of essential omega-3 fatty acid known to be cardio-protective, in the patients' blood by a phenomenal 80 percent.

The positive findings astonished Dr. Vuksan and his team. According to Dr. Vuksan, "These were huge discoveries rarely seen in medical literature, even with the most powerful and combined pharmacological therapies."

The study reported a six-unit drop in systolic blood pressure (the peak pressure in the arteries). "That's better than a lot of medications," Dr. Vuksan said.

High blood pressure is one of the most common health problems among people with diabetes and tends to amplify all of the disease's potential complications. According to Dr. Amir Hanna, who also worked on the study, "a six-unit blood pressure reduction would likely translate into less chance of cardiovascular events or kidney disease for a diabetes sufferer."

Dr. Vuksan has also been amazed with other findings from the study. "We measured the body inflammation, the so-called c-reactive protein, which has been discovered as a major risk factor for heart disease, even more important than cholesterol, according to studies from Harvard. This was one of the rarest studies in the world, showing that CRP dropped about 32 percent in type 2 diabetics who were heavily medicated and well controlled. The only other major studies showing a reduction in CRP have been done with statin drugs."

Dr. Vuksan measured another risk factor for cardiovascular disease, fibrinolytic factors. Fibrinogen is a type of protein, and recently health researchers have discovered when it is present in the blood in high levels, it can dramatically increase the risk of heart attack and other forms of heart disease. In addition, it can also multiply the risks of heart disease associated with other health hazards. That's because high blood levels of fibrinogen can significantly increase the likelihood of blood clots and other types of damage to the cardiovascular system.

Like cholesterol, fibrinogen is a naturally occurring substance in the body that plays an essential role in your body's overall health. In the case of fibrinogen, it is necessary for normal blood clotting that occurs in the body, such as in response to wounds. But when fibrinogen levels become higher than normal, they can cause abnormal blood clots to form, thereby making heart attacks, stroke, and other types of heart disease more likely.

In regards to fibrinolytic factors, Dr. Vuksan saw positive results. "The thickness of blood can determine heart problems. We actually found some of the major fibrinolytic factors, like factor VIII (linked to von

Willebrand's disease) and fibrinogen, were significantly reduced after Salba. We also measured bleeding time because, as you know, if you are thinning blood, you want to see whether the patient will bleed more. We measured three factors, and there was no change with Salba whatsoever. We concluded that basically Salba is a functional food that has a health yeffect in diabetic individuals."

As a scientist, Dr. Vuksan says this about Salba. "You simply don't see many other ingredients that can do what Salba can. You add this to any food, even bad food, and it will improve your health."

While the study results surprised researchers, they affirmed some ancient beliefs. Several centuries ago, runners were the chief means of communication for the Aztec civilization, and legend has it they subsisted on these seeds for days at a time. "It's now no wonder the Aztecs could run so long on this," Dr. Vuksan said. "Their circulation was better, their blood was thinner and their inflammation was less."

Dr. Vuksan's team wondered if some results were due to other nutrients hidden within Salba other than omega-3. They already knew from previous research that Salba's protein quality was higher than soy and it had the highest fiber content of any food. Upon further investigation, they realized Salba was a nutritional goldmine.

They calculated that 3 1/2 ounces of Salba contain as much calcium as 3 cups of milk, as much fiber as 1 1/4 cups of All-Bran cereal, as much iron as 5 cups of raw spinach, as much vegetable protein as 1 1/2 cups of kidney beans, as much potassium as 1 1/2 bananas, and as much vitamin C as seven oranges.

As a result of the many undisputed therapeutic benefits from consuming Salba, it has the distinction of being the only food that holds a pending medical patent (60-274.256). The patent pertains to Salba's ability to manage the effects of diabetes and the dietary approaches to such management.

CHAPTER FIVE

A UNIQUE FIBER SOLUTION

YOU PROBABLY KNOW YOUR WEIGHT. You may be a calorie, fat or carbohydrate counter. But do you even know why you might want to consider pondering your fiber intake? Or do you have any idea how many grams of fiber you should be eating each day?

For the vast majority of people, fiber doesn't make it on their radar. And when it comes to how much should be consumed, the answer is "not nearly enough" to reap all the benefits of the rough stuff, which include weight control, a lower risk of heart disease and diabetes and, of course, relief from constipation and other bowel ailments.

But fiber, far from the forgotten step-child of the nutritional world, is emerging as Cinderella...the belle of the ball! Both the American Cancer Society and the American Heart Association share the same message for those who may be fiber clueless - eat more high-fiber foods for cancer and heart protection.

A century ago, before the food supply became industrialized and highly processed, people ate a diet that included an average of 28 grams of fiber a day. Conditions such as diabetes, heart disease, and obesity were far less common then than they are now. Even today, in cultures that eat traditional, plant-based diets diabetes, cancer, and cardiovascular disease are still rare. By contrast, the United States currently ranks lowest in fiber intake and highest in deaths from heart disease among 20 developed nations.

In these days of plenty, just how much fiber are Americans eating? Just a pittance! The average adult consumes less than 12 grams of fiber per day (according to the U.S. Department of Agriculture). This is far short of the National Cancer Institute's healthy recommendation of 25 to 35 grams of fiber per day.

Studies of children's diets show similar shortfalls. Inadequate fiber intake may increase these children's risk of developing heart disease and other chronic illnesses later in life. According to the *Journal of the American Dietetic Association,* American preschool-age children are not making the grade when it comes to getting enough fiber from their diets.

The recommended dietary fiber intakes for children are:	
1 to 3 years:	19 grams
4 to 8 years:	25 grams
9–13 years:	26 grams (Female) 31 grams (Male)
14–18 years:	29 grams (Female) 38 grams (Male)

And it's no mystery why fiber intake is so low. Fiber – the indigestible part of plant-based foods – is plentiful in fruits, vegetables, whole grains, beans and nuts. The fiber component of food is known as dietary fiber. Our modern predilection for processed foods are sorely lacking is this important dietary constituent.

What is Dietary Fiber?

FIBER IS WHAT YOUR grandma used to call roughage. It's not one particular food but the part of plant foods your body can't digest. Fibers are technically carbohydrates but your body doesn't make the enzymes needed to break them down.

Fiber is divided into two basic types – insoluble and soluble. Foods differ in the type and amount of fiber they contain. But all types of fiber have two things in common: they are found only in plant foods and they are resistant to human digestive enzymes (that is they pass through the digestive tract without being completely broken down).

As a result fiber is not absorbed, provides no real nutrition and essentially has no calories.

But without adequate insoluble and soluble fiber in our diet, optimal health will continue to elude us.

Fiber Facts

INSOLUBLE FIBER (cellulose, hemicellulose, lignin) is what we would think of as roughage. It is a type of fiber that does not dissolve in water nor breaks down in your digestive system, thus contributing bulk and moisture to the stool. It passes through the intestines largely intact. It is estimated that 65 percent to 75 percent of dietary fiber in our diet is "insoluble."

Insoluble fiber is health-enhancing in the following ways.

* **Promotes regular bowel movements and prevents constipation**

* **Helps prevent hemorrhoids and varicose veins**

* **Removes toxic waste through colon in less time**

* **Helps prevent colon cancer (by keeping an optimal pH in intestines to prevent microbes from producing cancerous substances)**

* **Helps prevent the formation of gallstones (by binding with bile acids and removing cholesterol before stones can form)**

Insoluble fiber is found mainly in whole grains and on the outside of seeds, fruits, legumes, and other foods.

The other form of fiber is called soluble fiber (gums, mucilages, pectins). Soluble fiber retains water and turns into gel during digestion. While insoluble fiber absorbs water, resulting in bulkier, softer stool, soluble fiber ferments in the large intestine, producing short-chain fatty acids that significantly inhibit the development of invasive colon cancers.

Because soluble fiber absorbs readily into the body, it can be an effective tool in maintaining healthy blood sugar levels. Soluble fiber works to keep the rate of food passing through the system from progressing too quickly. This allows the nutrients derived from food to be efficiently absorbed into the system as well as creating a sense of fullness (which keeps you from getting hungry as quickly after a meal). Soluble fiber is thought to also help with maintaining healthy cholesterol levels, which may indirectly also promote a healthier cardiovascular system.

In addition, soluble fiber helps slow down digestion (which keeps you from getting hungry as quickly after a meal) and helps regulate blood sugar. A diet high in soluble fiber can help reduce your risk of heart disease, diabetes, and may help you lose weight.

Soluble fiber is found in fruits, vegetables, seeds, and, the bran of grains.

Why Fiber? For Six Good Reasons!

AS WE LEARN ABOUT the many benefits of the humble fiber, grandma, once again, is being proven right. Fiber is a must in our diet.

Fiber has always been known as nature's tool for cleaning the body and helping with the removal of toxins and waste. However, recent studies have revealed the numerous ways fiber plays an important role in a wide range of health issues.

1. Fiber promotes regularity by adding bulk to stool and stimulating the rapid movement of waste through the colon. By serving this purpose, fiber can help prevent bowel problems, including constipation and hemorrhoids.

Fiber also helps reduce the risk of diverticulosis, a condition in which small pouches form in the colon wall (usually from the pressure of straining during bowel movements). People who already have diverticulosis often find that increased fiber consumption can alleviate symptoms, which include constipation and/or diarrhea, abdominal pain, flatulence, and mucus or blood in the stool.

2. Fiber blocks the absorption of some of the dietary cholesterol and fat you eat, which can lower your numbers and help prevent plaque buildup that can lead to heart attack and stroke.

Fiber's ability to reduce the risk of developing and dying from coronary heart disease was among the earliest findings of dietary fiber research.

Fiber affects another heart disease risk factor known as C-reactive protein (CRP). Elevated CRP levels are associated with an increased risk of heart disease. A 2004 study by the federal Centers for Disease Control and Prevention examined the link between dietary fiber and CRP serum concentration. The researchers found that increased fiber intake was associated with lower levels of CRP. In fact, the risk of increased CRP concentration was almost halved for those with the highest fiber intake. Thus, fiber favorably influences numerous risk factors for cardiovascular disease, and may help to minimize or eliminate the need for potentially dangerous prescription drugs for cardiovascular health.

Dietary fiber also helps to reduce cholesterol by binding to cholesterol-laden bile excreted from the liver into the small intestine. This reduces the re-absorption of bile into the bloodstream and thus helps to lower total cholesterol, LDL, and serum triglyceride levels simultaneously.

3. Fiber protects against certain cancers, especially in the colon and rectum. Fiber helps "move things along" in the digestive tract, reducing the amount of time that stool is present in the intestinal tract. The less time it spends there, the less time bacteria have to metabolize it and produce substances that may act as carcinogens (cancer-causing agents).

A study conducted at the National Cancer Institute examined the relationship between the amount of fiber in the diet and the incidence of colorectal polyps, the precursors to colon cancer. It found that people who had the highest amounts of fiber in their diets (36 grams a day or more) had the lowest incidence of colon polyps. Their risk of getting polyps was 27 percent less than that of the people who ate the least amount of fiber (12 grams a day or less).

The researchers speculate that fiber may help lower risk by binding potential carcinogens and helping move waste through the colon more rapidly, giving harmful substances less time to damage the cells in the colon. Fiber also stimulates bacteria in the colon that produce compounds thought to slow cell proliferation that could lead to cancer.

But, it's not only colon cancer that can be reduced with fiber; fiber also improves lung function in chronic obstructive pulmonary disease (COPD). Individuals who consumed fiber had as much as a 28 percent lower risk. The researchers wrote, "This study provides the first known evidence that dietary fiber is independently associated with better lung function and reduced prevalence of COPD."

Studies also showed a relationship between high dietary fiber and reduced risk of pre-menopausal breast cancer. Fiber from cereals and potentially also from fruits may be the important sources of fiber resulting in this inverse relationship with pre-menopausal breast cancer.

In one U.K. study, women who ate 30g of fiber per day had half the risk of developing breast cancer in comparison to those who ate 20g or less.

In another study 213 women – all between 20 and 40 years old – were asked to eat either a high-fiber, low-fat diet, or their usual diet. The women also had their hormones levels tested. Over the year's time, the high fiber "healthy diet group" had an eight percent reduction in estrogen levels compared with the "regular diet" group that had less than a one percent drop.

In addition, dietary fiber intake has been shown to provide uterine cancer protection. A major meta-analysis published in the American *Journal of Clinical Nutrition* found that women consuming the highest amount of fiber had a 29 percent reduction in risk compared to women with the lowest average intake.

4. Fiber can lower fasting blood-sugar levels in diabetics and those at risk for diabetes, helping to reduce metabolic syndrome.

A recent article in the *Journal of Clinical Endocrinology & Metabolism* compared popular glycemic index-based, low-carbohydrate diets to a high-fiber, high-carbohydrate diet emphasizing fresh fruits and vegetables. The study findings suggest that the fiber content of the foods eaten – rather than their glycemic index – was most beneficial for promoting insulin sensitivity.

A classic Mediterranean diet, rich in carbohydrates and fiber from sources such as fruits, vegetables, whole grains, and nuts, has been shown over and over to be one of the best ways to improve metabolic syndrome. Because fiber slows the absorption of nutrients into the bloodstream, it naturally helps regulate blood sugar levels, preventing insulin surges and decreasing insulin resistance. It is abundantly clear the best way to manage metabolic syndrome and decrease all of the cardiovascular risks that accompany it is by eating a diet high in complex carbohydrates supplying at least 25 grams of fiber a day.

5. Fiber may also help you to achieve one thing almost everyone wants – weight loss. Not only does fiber help reduce calories by blocking fat absorption; it also acts as an appetite suppressant. The bulk provided by fiber is calorie-free and can make you feel full faster and longer than other foods. Controlling appetite is often one of the most difficult aspects of achieving weight loss, which is certainly a big plus for fiber.

Higher fiber intake is associated with lower average body weight in the US. In the Nurses Health Study, a prospective observational cohort study of female nurses without known chronic illnesses, those who ingested more dietary fiber consistently weighed less than those who consumed less fiber.

6. Fiber acts as a prebiotic. A prebiotic is something that feeds, or stimulates the growth of "good" bacteria in the gut and inhibits the growth of harmful bacteria. All fiber acts as a prebiotic, in varying degrees. By feeding our intestinal eco-system, fiber benefits our immunity and overall health.

Salba – A Superior Source of Fiber

THE BEST DIETARY FIBER comes from a whole-food plant based diet. The many health benefits of fiber were associated with eating the foods found in nature that contained high amounts of both soluble and insoluble fiber - not isolated fibers.

The complete nutrient package contributes to fiber's effectiveness. When fiber is part of a whole food that naturally contains a wide assortment of vitamins, minerals, essential fatty acids and antioxidants, it is able to deliver the best results.

When it comes to fiber, Salba is an excellent source. In fact, its rich fiber content is another reason why Salba is considered nature's perfect whole food.

One tablespoon of Salba seeds (12 g) contains 4.2 grams of dietary fiber – both insoluble and soluble. That's an impressive 17 percent of your daily requirement for fiber in just one tablespoon!

Salba Has More Fiber Than Flax

IF YOU'RE WONDERING how that compares with other fiber sources such as flax, gram for gram, Salba provides four times more fiber than flax. And besides higher fiber content, Salba's nutrient-dense profile is brimming over with high amounts of vitamins, minerals and antioxidants which are missing in flax seeds. Remember, it's the assortment of all those phyto-nutrients that adds the synergy to fiber's many health benefits.

Due to Salba's soluble fiber content, it is able to absorb up to 12 times its weight in water. That means when you add water or other liquids to it, it will expand in volume – a lot! In fact, Salba has the ability to absorb and hold more water than any other natural food. It can absorb twice the amount of water than flax seeds.

So, not only will Salba help to keep away those hunger pangs by creating a sense of fullness, its fiber will also help to balance your blood sugar and support healthy digestion and elimination. (Be sure to drink adequate amounts of water throughout the day.)

The rich insoluble fiber in Salba is most important for keeping the colon free of debris, physically "scrubbing" the walls so buildup does not occur reducing the risk of diverticulosis.

Adding Salba to other fiber rich foods such as whole grains, salads, fruits, stews, soups and baked goods will enable you to easily meet the daily recommended amount of the all-important 25-35 grams of fiber you and your family need to stay healthy.

Since Salba is such a user friendly food, it can also help children reach their daily fiber needs. Its neutral flavor allows it to be disguised by any food it is mixed with. So, add it to breakfast cereals, mix it into puddings or yogurt, include it in their favorite cookie recipe, or even sprinkle it into salads.

With the help of Salba, your daily fiber needs will always be met.

SALBA vs. FLAX

Flax seed is known primarily for its Omega-3 and Fiber composition. Here's a look at how Salba stacks up against flax on key nutrition statistics.

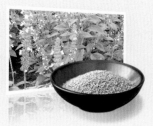 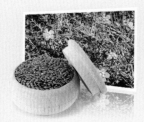

SALBA Multi-Dimensional Superfood	**FLAX** Omega-3 & Fiber Supplement
228.7mg of Omega-3s per Gram	**192.8mg of Omega-3s per Gram**
350.0mg of Fiber per Gram	**259.2mg of Fiber per Gram**
100% Non-Toxic; Safe for Use in Food Preparation	Contains Linamarin - A Toxic Cyanogenic Glycoside
Absorbs Between 8-12 Times its Weight in Water	Absorbs 6 Times its Weight in Water
Promotes an Alkaline Environment	Has an Acidic pH Level
100% Bioavailable & Convenient in Whole Seed Form	Thick Husk Must Be Ground to Release Omega-3s
Subtle, Neutral Flavor with No Bitter Aftertaste	Dominant Flavor with Bitter Aftertaste

*Based on USDA nutritional data.

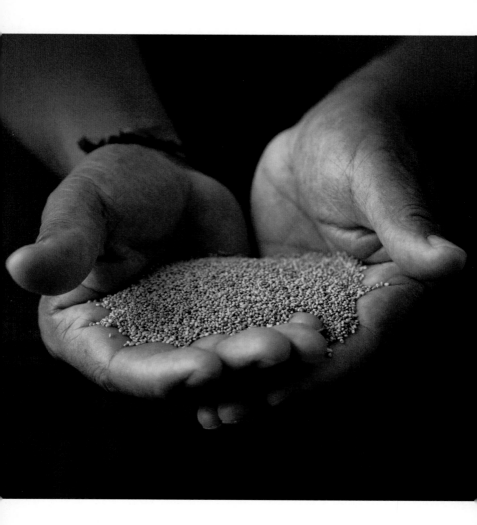

CHAPTER SIX

A KEY TO
FITNESS AND
ENERGY

WHATEVER ONE'S AGE – from childhood to seniorhood – physical energy and fitness are our most necessary requirements for living a vital life. It's not just the athlete that requires optimal energy. We all do. Whether it's running a marathon or running errands, without that current of life force pulsing through us, the zest for life just isn't there. Not only are we limited in what we can do and accomplish, lack of energy also dampens our moods and dulls our brain.

Our quality of life is really determined by our quality of energy. When our body is able to have a high energy output, we have the energy to heal, regenerate and repair our bodies. With an abundance of energy, we accomplish remarkable things.

Brendan Brazier is a living example of high-energy output. In 2003 and 2006 he won the grueling Canadian 50 km Ultra Marathon. As a professional Ironman tri-athlete, he knows all about the need for generating and sustaining energy. In order to achieve the best competitive edge, Brendan has been on a quest to discover the nutritional program for optimal energy. He realized the best performance and recovery rate was directly related to diet.

He began to experiment to find the best performance-enhancing diet. He tried high-carbohydrate, grain-based, low-fat, low-protein diets and low-carbohydrate, high-fat, high-protein diets…and several others that fell in-between. But none were able to give him the edge he was looking for. All this experimentation did result in one thing – he became an even stronger believer in the powerful effect nutrition has on the body.

On a mission to accomplish his goal of optimal health and vitality as well as winning athlete, he did the unthinkable for an athlete - he focused on developing a plant-based diet that would be based on high-quality, nutrient-dense, alkaline-forming, easily digestible food. His decision defied conventional athletic wisdom: a professional Ironman tri-athlete eating a plant-based diet? Impossible!

His winning performance in two Ironman competitions proved all the experts wrong.

After much research not only from nutritional experts but also from experimenting with his own body, he devised a vegetarian program that enabled him to recover at an unprecedented rate. By paying detailed attention to his diet, his body was able to adapt to his intensive trainings with remarkable speed. And he began to win his Ironman events.

But on his journey to become the best athlete he could possibly be, Brendan discovered something even more important. On a cellular level, his diet was able to speed the renewal of muscle tissue. That meant it could actually help the body to regenerate.

The stress incurred from strenuous exercise reduces the body's ability to recover. The more stress, the slower recovery time. Brendan realized a plant-based diet i.e. better nutrition, had a huge impact on the body's response to stress. Since stress is a major component of all chronic illness, the implication that this diet could make a big dent in stress levels for all people not just athletes was significant.

Brendan's experiment with diet became the basis of his program called the Thrive Diet and is described in detail in his book "The Thrive Diet: The Whole Food Way to Lose Weight, Reduce Stress, and Stay Healthy for Life". He extols the health benefit of this program not just for high-level athletes but also for all people no matter their activity level. He believes by helping to reduce nutritional stress and thus overall stress, the Thrive Diet can potentially eliminate up to 40 percent of total stress on the average North American's body.

Nutritional stress is the term used to describe the body's response to food that is totally void of nutrition and/or foods that require a large amount of energy to digest and assimilate – unrefined, unnatural ones.

Understanding High-Net-Gain Foods

THE CORNERSTONE of Brendan's program is based on the concept of high net-gain foods. He explains the concept:

"The net-gain of food is the term I have given to the energy and usable sustenance we are left with once digestion and assimilation have taken place. As you know, the body gets energy from food in the form of several nutrients. However, the more energy the body has to expend to digest, assimilate and utilize the nutrients in the food we give it, the less we are left with. As mentioned earlier, *The Thrive Diet* was designed to reduce stress. For nutritional stress to be minimized, efficiency of digestion and nutrient assimilation must be maximized. Essentially what high net gain eating does is eliminates excess work for the body to perform."

What was the key to Brendan's ability to gain and maintain strength, lean muscle and have an abundance of energy for high performance training while eating fewer calories than most? Stop counting calories and start "net-gain" eating.

"Instead of feasting on common refined foods, I now consume whole foods almost exclusively. Raw, alkalizing, enzyme-intact foods have become the foundation of my diet."

Salba - A Perfect Net-Gain Food

THE CONSUMPTION OF nutrient–dense foods reduces the stress response and allows the body to conserve energy to be used as fuel and building blocks.

Always on the lookout for the best nutrient-dense foods available, Brendan recognized what a phenomenal food Salba was for his program.

"Salba offers a more seed-like nutritional profile. A higher percentage of protein, more fiber and richer in trace minerals than grains and it is also gluten free.

Packed with antioxidants and comprised of about 20 percent high-quality protein, Salba is extremely nutrient-dense and digests easily. Therefore, its net gain is exceptionally high. Particularly rich in magnesium, potassium, calcium and iron Salba can effectively replenish minerals used in muscle contractions and lost in sweat. Additionally, Salba can promote smooth and effortless muscle movement, thereby reducing the amount of work required for each contraction. This is significant. Increased muscle efficacy directly translates to improved athletic performance. Salba is also high in both soluble and insoluble fiber, which helps to sustain energy and maintain fullness. Very versatile, Salba can be used to replace up to 20 percent of the flour in baking, packing it with nutrition."

As a perfect energy food, Salba has a lot more going for it. In addition to being rich in antioxidants and electrolytes, it is also easily digested. As a nutrient-dense whole food Salba is gluten-free which means anyone who is gluten-intolerant or suffers from Celiac disease can add it safely to his or her diet. And of course, it is non-GMO, which is turning out to be another important feature for any truly healthy food. (Learn more about the problem of GMO foods at www. seadsofdeception.com.)

Salba - A High Quality Protein

FOR THOSE WHO ARE ON high protein diets, Salba provides 95 percent of its calories from high quality plant protein (21 percent) and from Omega 3's (74 percent) with very few calories from carbohydrates. The carbohydrate portion of Salba is predominantly insoluble fiber. Insoluble fiber, which is very beneficial to digestion, is a "non-carbohydrate" carbohydrate that passes through the gastro-intestinal tract undigested resulting in a non-caloric effect to our body.

The proteins in Salba show an excellent distribution of amino acids, including all essential amino acids. Calculation of the Protein Efficiency Ratio (PER) indicates that Salba protein has a digestibility in the range of other proteins used in nutritional products of the highest standard. The PER for Salba is slightly lower than that of casein, a skim milk protein and a standard of comparison of protein quality. However, it is slightly higher than that of soy protein, a common and highly regarded source of quality protein.

Protein quality is the estimated percentage of protein that is likely to be used by the body. Protein quality calculations yield relative protein quality for Salba of 91 percent and for flax of 60 percent (both based on limiting value, Lysine). - Salba has 1.5 to two times the protein concentration of other common grains.

Salba Reduces Lactic Acid Build-up

EVER FEEL A BURN in your muscles during exercise? What you are experiencing is a build-up of lactic acid in your muscles.

With physical exertion, especially in sports-related activities, lactic acid build-up can occur in the muscles and possibly cause cramping or burning. To help with the body's post exercise repair process, it is essential to alkaline the body by eating alkalizing foods. If not addressed, the build-up of lactic acid from physical exertion, general stress and acid-forming foods will lead to muscular stiffness, fatigue and joint pain.

Salba can help with the effects of lactic acid buildup in several ways. First of all, it is an alkaline-forming food, helping to maintain the proper pH of the body. A sign we are excessively acidic is the build-up of lactic acid.

In addition, Salba contains many of the minerals that are lost through sweating (these minerals are also known as electrolytes) such as: potassium, magnesium, iron and phosphorus. Since Salba is so mineral-rich, it is a much-preferred alternative to the less-than-healthy popular electrolyte replacements such as Gatorade.

Salba is a very special complex carbohydrate generally taking 3.5 to four hours to digest. This slower digestion period keeps the body hydrated longer, allowing you to fully absorb all of its valuable nutrients, and dramatically increasing energy and endurance.

Salba is also a hydrophilic colloid (a watery, gelatinous, substance which forms the underlying elements of all living cells). This means when it is mixed with water, it is able to absorb its weight many times over. In fact, it is able to hold eight times its weight in water thereby offering prolonged cellular hydration.

This important property aids in the digestion of food and helps control excess acids associated with indigestion, heartburn, sour stomach, and ulcers.

Salba Fresca

DURING THE hot Mexican summer, the locals have a favorite drink made with *Salvia hispanica* seeds,. They are soaked in water with added lemon juice (and sugar to taste). This is not only a refreshing drink but it also essential to help maintain proper hydration.

Thus, Salba is especially beneficial for athletes who need to remain hydrated during races and endurance activities.

You can make your own version of this drink, called Salba Fresca. Try adding one or two tablespoons of Salba in a glass or water or juice and let it sit for about 15 minutes before drinking. It will turn into a gel consistency. Stir gently and add lemon or lime juice to taste. You can drink it before, during or after strenuous exercise.

Whether a cooling drink to sip on during a hot day or a hydrating beverage to take with you while exercising, a Salba drink is an effective way to replace vital electrolytes and restore healthy cellular hydration.

Salba – A New Version of the Ancient Running Food

THE HUMBLE ORIGINS of Salba were from seeds traditionally eaten by the ancient Aztecs and southwest Native Americans. It was said the Indians would eat as little as a teaspoon when going on a 24-hour forced march. As we learn more about Salba, it has become evident why the ancient athletes, as well as modern-day athletes, would rely on such a perfect running food.

Salba Supports Physical Activity and Recovery

SALBA IS THE IDEAL FOOD that supports the body's needs during times of increased physical activity.

SALBA vs. SOY

The soybean has earned a lofty reputation as the definitive vegetarian source of protein. Here's how Salba measures up to this time-tested super food.

Salba has 70% more quality protein than Soy.

Salba has a neutral, thus a more appealing flavor.

Salba has almost 10 times more Omega 3's than Soy.

Salba has more fiber than Soy.

Salba has more calcium than Soy.

Salba has more potassium than Soy.

Salba has a superior micro-nutrient composition.

Salba is easy to digest: Soy is difficult to digest.

Salba is non-GMO; Soy is one of the four major gene-modified crops.

Salba has clinical studies demonstrating its effect on blood pressure, body inflammation or blood thinning in Type 2 Diabetes: Soy has none.

Salba's clinically proven reduction of inflammatory markers increases physical performance and accelerates sports recovery

In addition to its high mineral and vitamins content, Salba's extraordinary amounts of Omega 3's provide sustained energy as well as anti-inflammatory benefits. Salba's clinically proven reduction of inflammatory markers and high protein efficiency ratio helps regenerate muscle tissue and accelerates sports recovery.

One of the side effects of any form of exercise is the production of free radicals. It just goes with the exercising territory. Also, with its high ORAC value, Salba's antioxidants help to combat the increased free radicals produced not only from strenuous exercise but also from stress, in general.

Once in the stomach, Salba turns into a mucilaginous, gel-like substance, which creates a physical barrier between carbohydrates and the digestive enzymes that break them down. This process slows the conversion of carbohydrates into sugar. This stabilization of blood sugar is just what is needed to generate sustained endurance.

With Salba's high protein efficiency ratio, muscle tissue can be regenerated.

Whether you are a high performance athlete or someone who enjoys a walk around the block, we all need to be eating foods that are rich in the fundamental nutritional requirements of the body i.e. minerals, vitamins, essential fatty acids, antioxidants, protein and fiber. Fueling the body with superior nutrition is the key to achieving peak performance for all of life's activities.

CHAPTER SEVEN

A SUPERIOR
GLUTEN FREE
SOLUTION

FROM A DIETARY PERSPECTIVE, Western cultures have a love affair with grains, especially wheat. Americans wax lyrical about their "amber waves of grain". And when it comes to wheat products, they are about as American as…well, apple pie.

What would life be like without our hot dog rolls, Wheaties, pizzas, pancakes, brownies, cookies, crackers, pretzels, cakes, licorice, breads, and muffins?

But, along the way something has happened to the nature of wheat and other grains that contain gluten (the storage proteins gliadin and prolamine). The humble grain that many of our ancestors ate has been transformed through hybridization, genetic engineering and selective breeding into a very different kind of grain. In addition, modern farming and storage practices routinely spray pesticides, insecticides and fungicides throughout a seed's life cycle – from sowing to harvesting to grain elevator storage. This all adds up to a food the cells in our digestive system can barely recognize as digestible. In fact, it turns out that gluten is one of the hardest proteins for the human system to digest.

In addition to wheat, gluten is found in barley, rye, kamut, spelt and triticale. The gluten problem is even more complicated since gluten can be a hidden ingredient in many products. It can be found in a large variety of foods including soups, salad dressings, processed foods and natural flavorings. It can also lurk in unidentified starch, binders and fillers in medications or vitamins.

The body's reaction to foods such as gluten products creates what is known as delayed food response or intolerance. Unlike true allergies, which produce immediate histamine responses with itching or hives, a delayed food response can present itself in a variety of unsuspecting ways from two hours to three days after the consumption of the culprit food.

What causes an intolerance or sensitivity? It is the result of the gut lining immunity reacting to a certain food type. The gut lining then becomes irritated and inflamed. This condition can be occurring for years, if not decades, before obvious symptoms appear. It is a continuous inflammatory condition that, unbeknownst to most people, is compromising overall health.

Once the gut lining becomes damaged, particles of food, which should not be able to reach the bloodstream, start to breach the gut lining. This is the origin of the kind of allergies, which inconvenience most people. Undigested food particles in the bloodstream are treated as a foreign bodies and the immune system develops an antibody to attack them.

The distress this causes to the body stimulates the release of adrenocorticotropic hormone, better known as ACTH, which stimulates the adrenal glands to produce more cortisol, the long-term stress hormone.

This causes strain on the adrenal and thyroid glands and also triggers a vicious circle because high cortisol levels also irritate the gut lining.

For many people, the daily consumption of common foods, such as those containing gluten, may actually be the portal to life-long health problems that undermine optimal health.

On the extreme end of the gluten intolerance spectrum is a genetic autoimmune disease called Celiac disease, a life-long inflammatory disease of the upper small intestine. The gluten proteins damage the small finger-like projections (villi) that line the small intestine resembling a pile in a carpet. When damaged and inflamed, the villi are unable to absorb water and nutrients such as vitamins, folic acid, iron and calcium. This causes the celiac to be susceptible to a variety of other conditions related to malabsorption.

For a person diagnosed with Celiac disease, consuming any gluten foods is simply not an option. It's like waving a red flag to the gut. The healing process requires the lifelong excommunication of all gluten containing foods. Even small amounts of gluten can trigger an inflammatory response.

"Celiac disease is not just a disease of the gut," says Shelley Case, R.D., nutrition consultant and author of *Gluten Free Diet: A Comprehensive Resource Guide*. "It's a multi-system, multi-symptom disease with serious implications."

Celiac disease is linked to malnutrition that can lead to anemia, osteoporosis, depression, behavioral problems, and stunted growth in children, among other problems. Some of the autoimmune diseases associated with Celiac disease are Type 1 Diabetes, Rheumatoid Arthritis, Jorgen's Syndrome, Autoimmune Thyroid Disease (Hashimoto's Thyroiditis), Crohn's Disease, Multiple Sclerosis, as well as others. Researchers recently found that diabetes and thyroid related antibodies in Celiac disease patients disappeared after the patient is put on a gluten free diet.

Researchers are also beginning to see a connection between gluten and other disorders, which seem to share characteristics such as biochemical, neurological, and immunological abnormalities. These "Overlapping Syndromes" are conditions such as Gulf War Syndrome, Chronic Fatigue Syndrome, and Fibromyalgia Syndrome, as well as others. Also, some psychological disorders such as depression and panic disorder as well as skin conditions such as psoriasis are suspected to have a gluten-related component.

It is becoming apparent the problem of gluten sensitivity is far greater than most people have ever realized. Presently one in 133 people have some form of Celiac disease. Among those with parents, siblings, or children with Celiac disease, up to one in 22 people may have it. As many as three million Americans have Celiac disease. Most of them don't know it, largely because Celiac disease can be difficult to properly diagnose.

Many doctors believe that gluten intolerance in an unrecognized health epidemic. Upwards of 70 percent of Americans have inherited a genetic tendency for gluten sensitivity, and experts estimate about half of the general population has some degree of it. Dr. Joseph Mercola, best-selling author, ostepathic physician and health activist, suggests gluten intolerance is a very common condition that affects a considerable proportion of the population. "Recent research has put the figure as high as one in every 33 people, but my experience tells me that it is more like one in every 10 people. (http://www.mercola.com/2000/aug/6/wheat_miscarriage.htm)

Specific Symptoms of Gluten Intolerance and Celiac Disease:

* **Weight loss or weight gain**
* **Nutritional deficiencies due to malabsorption e.g. low iron levels**
* **Gastro-intestinal problems (bloating, pain, gas, constipation, diarrhea)**
* **Fat in the stools**
* **Aching joints, arthritis, muscle aches**
* **Depression**
* **Eczema**
* **Headaches**
* **Exhaustion**
* **Irritability and behavioral changes**
* **Infertility, irregular menstrual cycle and miscarriage**
* **Cramps, tingling and numbness**
* **Slow infant and child growth**
* **Panic attacks, ADD, irritability, nervousness**
* **Decline in dental health**
* **Mucus problems i.e. congested nose and sinuses, persistent phlegm**
* **Yo-yoing weight and edema**

Autism, ADD and Gluten –Intolerance

GLUTEN INTOLERANCE is now being associated with Autistic Spectrum Disorders and Attention Deficit Disorders. The type of gluten intolerance associated with these conditions is considered to originate from the body's inability to break down the gluten and casein proteins rather than an autoimmune response, as in Celiac disease.

For most Autistic children, gluten and casein are the equivalent of poison. This is not because of allergies, but because many of these children are unable to properly break down these proteins. They leak into the gut, undigested, and attach to the opiate receptors of the autistic's brain. Essentially, many autistic children are "drugged" on wheat and milk products, as if they were on a morphine drip.

A study by the University of California Davis Health System found that children with autism born in the 1990s were more likely to have gastrointestinal problems, including constipation, diarrhea and vomiting, than autistic children who were born in the early 1980s

It is recommended that every autistic child be placed on a gluten-free, casein-free diet for at least three months.

A Celiac's Story

KEITH IS A TYPICAL GUY. It takes a lot to get him to pay attention to his health…and even more to do something about it. Looking back he now recognizes he has been gluten sensitive since childhood. But for his first 38 years, he managed to lead a successful busy life in spite of bouts of fatigue, indigestion, some aches here and there and bouts of diarrhea. His condition was sub-clinical. A problem is brewing but it is not chronic enough to create serious health problems.

Keith should have suspected he had a problem with gluten intolerance since both his mother and aunt had been diagnosed years earlier with Celiac disease. However, he basically chose to ignore things.

Eventually, the time finally arrived when he could no longer deny the reality he had a serious problem. His health seemed to be going downhill fast. "I started having horrible chronic diarrhea on a daily basis and, on top of that, it was really foul smelling." Keith also felt constantly debilitated, dehydrated and exhausted. He especially noticed his symptoms became more intense right after he would consume gluten-containing foods.

Keith finally realized it was time

to seek advice from his doctor. As he suspected, the diagnosis was Celiac disease. It was a life changing moment. "The diagnosis empowered me right away." He began to take charge of his life that included making important lifestyle changes. Keith found effective ways to handle his stress and also found a supportive organization, the Gluten Intolerance Group (www.gluten.net) to help initiate him into this new gluten-free world.

As a Celiac, foods with gluten are forbidden forever! Any amount of gluten - no matter how small - will exacerbate inflammatory response.

Keith made the decision he would manage his disease by going the nutritional route rather than relying on medications.

While searching for healthy food options, Keith discovered Salba. He began by regularly including at least 2 or more tablespoons into his diet. He soon discovered Salba was a lifesaver!

The daily consumption of Salba helped Keith's body to heal. It was not long after starting to using Salba he noticed his stools were firmer, a major indicator of positive change for a Celiac sufferer. But the biggest change was his renewed energy. "I finally had sustained energy levels when I consistently used two tablespoons of Salba daily."

Keith also attributes Salba for his increased joint mobility. His constant achiness disappeared. Keith was also surprised by another unexpected benefit: the disappearance of pain from a rotator cuff injury.

The Gluten Solution - Let Me Count the Ways

SALBA IS AN IDEAL SOLUTION for anyone with any kind of gluten issue whether it's mild gluten sensitivity or a more full-blown auto-immune condition like Celiac disease.

First and foremost, the reason why Salba fulfills the number one criteria for anyone dealing with a gluten intolerance issue is because it is certified 100 percent gluten-free.

People with gluten issues have another serious health challenge to contend with - severe malabsorption and malnourishment. Since their digestive tract is so inflamed and the ability to absorb nutrients is so compromised, they cannot properly absorb and assimilate the nutrition from their diet. Salba provides extraordinary nutrient-density with its complete assortment of important vitamins, minerals, anti-oxidants, fiber (both soluble and insoluble) and protein. For this reason, even the most digestively impaired person, whether it's the elderly, someone convalescing from a serious illness or surgery, or children with autism (who are known to be gluten intolerant) will benefit from Salba.

People with gluten intolerances have chronic inflammation. Salba's high content of the anti-inflammatory Omega-3 essential fatty acids (Salba is the richest vegetarian source of EFAs in nature) is the perfect healing food to reduce the inflammation of those with gluten-intolerance.

Another unique feature of Salba is its neutral flavor. Since it doesn't really have a distinctive taste, it is easily disguised when mixed with other foods. A child on the autistic spectrum can have many contributing factors that can lead to extreme food selectivity where nutrition and health issues arise.

Extreme food selectivity is well beyond the scope of what parents would call fussy eating - it implies the eating of very small quantities of food and/or only eating from a very limited range of foods. Salba successfully may be added to or cooked with foods that are acceptable to these children. The seeds can be sprinkled directly onto foods or ground and mixed into other dishes. Salba can also be made into a gel by dissolving it in water or other liquids and then included as an ingredient. As a form of stealth nutrition, Salba can help provide the missing nutrition these children desperately need.

There is one final reason why Salba is an ideal food for all people – with or without gluten sensitivities. Salba is grown in mineral-rich soils without any pesticides or insecticides. Therefore it is totally free of the chemicals that are known to be toxic contaminants that contribute to gut irritation and inflammation.

Keith was so delighted with the contribution Salba has made to his health and healing he now describes himself as a lifelong Salba devotee. "Salba's total nutrition, in addition to being a great gluten-free food has provided me a way to replace taking lots of supplements."

It's understandable why Keith is such a Salba fan - it changed his life! "Salba is what I would call a great one stop solution that is easy for someone. It is not only convenient and easy to use but it also has a great versatility as an ingredient that can be incorporated into just about any recipe."

It's Official – Salba is Certified Gluten Free

THE MISSION of the Gluten Intolerance Group of North America (GIG) is to provide support to persons with gluten intolerances, including Celiac disease, and other gluten sensitivities, in order to live healthy lives.

GIG emerged out of the need to help the millions of people dealing with some degree of gluten intolerance to access more knowledge and safe food choices as well as providing a host of other services and programs including on-going support groups nation-wide, a GIG Kids Camp programs, gluten-free recipes, the Gluten-Free Restaurant Awareness Program (GFRAP), an annual education conference, and an advocacy group. It also has an extensive list of free educational publications for download from its website (http://www.gluten.net).

In order to ensure people can be guaranteed food is gluten free, GIG has created the only gluten-free cert-ification program in the world. If a product tests for less than 10 parts per million (the FDA standard is less than 20 parts per million), it has qualified as gluten-free and can display the GIG's Gluten Free logo. Products carrying the GF logo represent unmatched reliability and for meeting strict gluten-free standards.

Cynthia Kupper, the Executive Director of GIG and someone who has, herself, been diagnosed with Celiac disease has personally benefited from Salba.

She is not hesitant about praising Salba's many benefits. "Salba is a fabulous nutritional supplement for persons with gluten intolerances. It offers an easily digested fiber source, antioxidants, omega 3 and 6. It can easily be substituted for gums in gluten free products, allowing you to add nutrition easily to your food."

Salba is proud to have been certified by GIG and is approved to display the GF Logo on its packaging. This is just one of many validations reinforcing the fact that Salba is indeed, the superior gluten-free alternative.

CHAPTER EIGHT

SALBA
FOOD FOR LIFE LONG VITALITY

THERE IS A SAYING THAT GOES "Genes load the gun but the environment pulls the trigger." This refers to the fact the exposure to environmental toxins plays a significant role in determining whether certain genetic mutations will occur. This daring thought has challenged the world of genetics.

If external influences can alter gene expression in a negative way, can the opposite occur? If we were to change our external environment in some positive manner, can our genes then be affected positively?

The theory of genetic determinism, which taught the genes we were born with are the final arbiters of our destiny, has been replaced with another emerging understanding. Far from being fixed and predetermined, it has now been proven, genes can be altered to either turn on or off their expression in a number of ways.

If external influences can alter gene expression in a negative way, can the opposite occur? If we were to change our external environment in some positive manner, can our genes then be affected positively?

The answer to this important question is an emphatic "Yes!" As it turns out, one of the most powerful influences on gene expression happens to be food, or more specifically nutrition. Far beyond the obvious purpose of food, which is to provide nourishment to all our cells, it turns out wholesome food has the power within our bodies to profoundly alter gene expression. This frontier is called Nutrigenomics, the science of nutrition and genetics.

Ruth DeBusk, a geneticist, registered dietitian and author of *Genetics: The Nutrition Connection* heads an international coalition determined to educate experts — as well as the general public — about the benefits of nutrigenomics on over-all health and longevity. "Genes represent the blueprint for who we are, but they are not a jail sentence. They are not set in stone. Yes, the genes you inherit influence your health, but you can change the outcome and have greater control on how healthy you can be."

A recent study led by Dr. Dean Ornish, head of the Preventative Medicine Research Institute in California, produced astonishing results on the influence of diet and lifestyle on genes (*Proceedings of the National Academy of Sciences, June 2008*). It showed that comprehensive lifestyle changes incorporating a healthy diet and exercise could lead not only to a better physique, but also to swift and dramatic changes at the genetic level. The researchers tracked 30 men with low-risk prostate cancer. The men underwent three months of major lifestyle changes, including eating a diet rich in fruits, vegetables, whole grains, legumes along with moderate exercise such as walking for half an hour a day, and an hour of daily stress management methods such as meditation.

As expected, they lost weight, lowered their blood pressure and saw other health improvements. But the researchers found more profound changes when they compared prostate biopsies taken before and after the lifestyle changes.

After just three months, the men had changes in the activity in about 500 genes. The activity of disease-preventing genes increased while a number of disease-promoting genes, including those involved in prostate cancer and breast cancer, shut down.

Genes may be our predisposition but they're not our fate. Dr. Ornish hopes the findings may motivate people who think there's nothing they can do. According to Dr. Ornish, "It's an exciting finding because so often people say, 'Oh, it's all in my genes, what can I do?' Well, it turns out you may be able to do a lot. In just three months, I can change hundreds of my genes simply by changing what I eat and how I live. That's pretty exciting."

Perhaps the most surprising thing about the study is not the men changed their genetic profiles, but that they changed them so quickly – in just three months.

According to Dr. Ornish, "The implications of our study are not limited to men with prostate cancer." Similar outcomes can also be applied to other cancers and health conditions…and even aging itself.

Listen to the Health Experts

It may be no surprise nutritious foods play a major role in helping to repair, regenerate and detoxify our cells. However, it is quite mind-boggling to realize the food we choose to eat can directly impact our genes and the time it takes to affect our genes can be a little as three months.

Food truly is our best medicine and the cornerstone for lifelong vitality.

And Salba is in the forefront of providing the full spectrum of essential nutrients required to feed all the cells of our body as well as ensuring healthy gene expression.

A new paradigm is emerging in the world of traditional medicine. Instead of relying totally on drugs as the first line of defense, nutrition, as well as lifestyle, is now recognized as the foundation for restoring health.

Thomas Lodi, M.D.

Homeopathic Physician, Integrative Oncology, Certified Nutrition Specialist, Founder of An Oasis for Healing Center for Comprehensive Cancer Care

Dr. Thomas Lodi has been practicing medicine for 22 years. For the first ten years of his medical career, Dr. Lodi worked in conventional settings as an internal medicine specialist, urgent care physician, and as an intensivist in ICU and CCU departments of various hospitals. Subsequently, Dr Lodi continued his search for more effective and less toxic therapies by training around the world from Japan to Europe to Mexico and all around the U.S.

Although he occasionally sees patients with a variety of medical conditions, Dr. Lodi has narrowed his scope of practice through specific training and extensive experience over the past 12 years to Integrative Oncology (caring for people with cancer).

Dr. Lodi's main area of practice is alternative cancer treatment. In 2005 he established An Oasis for Healing in Mesa, Arizona. The foundation of the program at An Oasis for Healing is restoring the integrity of the immune system and organ function through detoxification and proper nutrition.

Proper nutrition is a key component to Dr. Lodi's comprehensive program. He not only incorporates an organic raw food diet as part of his treatment protocol but also teaches his patients how to stop cancer from recurring by living a raw foods lifestyle.

Since wholesome raw foods are a critical part of the healing program, Dr. Lodi has included Salba into his dietary protocol. He is particularly impressed with the high Omega-3 content since cancer patients really need to reduce inflammation and restore the health and function of cell membranes. His patients eat at least four tablespoons of Salba every day.

Dr. Lodi strongly believes Salba is "the most complete source of a lipid package in one product by nature for humans. I recommend Salba for everyone, not just cancer patients. As far as I'm concerned, 'seeds are it.' They have so much life force and are packed with key nutrients for human health."

(Dr. Lodi's raw food recipes with Salba can be found in the Chapter 9 – Salba Recipes.)

Michelle Hemingway, M.D.

One such doctor, who had adopted this paradigm shift, is Michelle Hemingway, M.D. who practices Integral Medicine in Lenox, Massachusetts. Integral medicine encompasses the whole human being – body, mind and spirit. It also integrates the best of what medical science has to offer with the wisdom of holistic modalities.

Dr. Hemingway believes in the importance of nutrition for health and longevity. According to Dr. Hemingway, "Nutrition is everything. So many health problems are related to poor nutrition – from eating too many of the bad foods."

When she was first introduced to Salba, she recognized it was a perfect addition to her nutritional program. While she recommends Salba to most of her patients, she especially encourages her diabetic patients as well as her patients with inflammatory issues to eat Salba. In her practice, Dr. Hemingway has experienced Salba's powerful blood sugar balancing ability as well as its anti-inflammatory effects.

Dr. Hemingway advises the use of both the Salba seeds as well as the Salba oil. "The seeds offer complete nutrition and are so versatile as an ingredient in the diet. It can easily be added to many foods and dishes. Lots of people sprinkle the seeds directly onto their salads and cereals because they like the crunchy texture. I also love the Salba oil because it is high in Omega 3's and is so much more stable than flax seed oil. My patients really like the taste and benefits from Salba."

Kasis Rote, D.C.

Another health practitioner that has become a Salba fan is Kasi Rote D.C., the founder of Rote Wellness, an alternative health clinic offering natural approaches to health in Dallas Texas. Dr. Rote integrates bioenergetic and chiropractic techniques with clinical nutrition, diet and lifestyle correction.

Dr. Rote specializes in difficult or "impossible" cases that have not responded well to other treatment (either medical or alternative). She has found that getting results on these difficult cases is possible because of the vast power of the body to heal itself. She believes her job "is to get the stops out of the way so the body is free to heal."

Nutrition plays a fundamental part of her healing program. Dr. Rote loves Salba because it is a powerful source of complete nutrition that has an impact on energy, vitality, and overall health. Its high quality omega 3 essential fatty acids and fiber help to reduce inflammation and a feeling of hunger, helping with weight loss.

For Dr. Rote it is important her patients follow a gluten-free diet, even if a patient is not gluten intolerant. She has found eating gluten foods such as wheat can increase fluid retention, adding to weight gain. As a gluten-free food, Salba can be incorporated as an ingredient in to many recipes replacing the need for gluten grains.

Recent studies have found eating a potassium rich diet will help older adults preserve muscle mass (*U.S. Department of Agriculture 2008, May 27 Foods For Preserving Muscle Mass 2008*). The study found increased potassium from the diet could help reduce the muscle mass loss older adults 65 and over experience -- approximately 4.4 pounds in a ten year span. Strong muscle mass reduces the risk of falls and injuries from damaged muscles.

Through her diagnostic techniques, Dr. Rote has found that a potassium deficiency (especially in relationship to sodium) has contributed to cellular dehydration, which reduces the body's ability to develop muscle mass.

Potassium-plentiful foods consist of a wide spectrum of raw vegetables and fruits. Amongst the many minerals found in Salba, it is a particularly rich source of potassium. This is another reason why Dr. Rote thinks Salba is such a phenomenal food for her patients. It helps to establish the proper potassium/sodium ratio of 5:1, which is necessary to restore cellular hydration. She has found many of her patients actually have the reverse 1:5 ratio of potassium to sodium. This results in too much intercellular sodium causing the cells to become dehydrated.

Gram for gram, Salba has more potassium than what is found in a banana, which is a high-potassium food. The potassium in Salba, in combination with all of its other important minerals and nutrients, can also help to maintain healthy blood pressure, proper kidney function, ease leg and muscle cramps and strengthen energy levels.

Marybeth Keener, LMT, CCH, AADP

Another health practitioner that has made Salba an intrinsic part of her nutritional program is Marybeth Keener. It was a chronic health challenge that eventually led Marybeth to the world of complementary health care over a decade ago. After a full year of conventional Western medicine treatments failed to resolve her own health care crisis, she turned to nutritional therapy, exercise, stress reduction techniques and therapeutic massage. When these approaches brought her improvement within three months - and an eventual return to wellness - Marybeth decided to become a practitioner of complementary health care modalities.

Marybeth established her healing center, Wellness Through Balance, in Glastonbury, Connecticut, a successful complementary medicine practice specializing in nutrition, exercise, acupuncture, massage therapies and stress reduction.

Nutrition is also a foundation of her practice. Since discovering Salba several years ago, it has now become an important part of the nutritional protocol for her patients. Salba has helped so many of her patients regain their health.

"As a nutritional biochemist, I am always looking for new whole foods that my clients can incorporate into their diet. With Salba many people found they received increased energy, less blood sugar swings, and better moods. There was even a marked glow to the women's skin - wrinkles were also less visible as Salba's EFAs plumped up their skin! I heartily recommend it to all my clients now. It seems to help with low level depression (especially the Seasonal Affective Disorder so many Northerners experience during winter), food cravings and increase sports stamina."

She has seen some impressive results with chronic health issues. "Salba is great for skin problems such as eczema and psoriasis. Its high Omega-3 content really does help to heal the skin. A friend's husband has been seeing a dermatologist for ten years. After just two months of using Salba, his psoriasis totally cleared up."

She believes that Salba should be included in the diet of teenagers and children. "The fiber and Omega 3's in Salba can help teenagers improve their complexion and even clear up acne. Teenagers just don't eat enough nutritious food. Children with sensitive stomachs and food allergies also do really well on Salba. Because it is essentially tasteless, it can be slipped into all sorts of foods and you can even bake with it. It a great food for those kids who are picky eaters because they don't even know it's there."

Jodi Hutchinson
Physician's Assistant, Health Coach

Jodi Hutchinson is part of a health team at the Center for Integrative Health associated with the Christiana Care Hospital in Delaware. As a health coach, Jodi guides and encourages her patients to make the best nutritional and life style choices to support their wellbeing.

Eating a wholesome diet is fundamental to recovering from any illness. Although, Jodi was impressed with the nutrient profile of Salba, it was one of her patient's extraordinary experience with Salba that really opened her eyes to its nutritional power.

A 62-year old woman with a history of cardiomyopathy, a serious heart condition arrived at the health center. Her heart function, which should have been around 55 percent, was only limping along at 18 percent. Her condition was caused by a virus that attacked and weakened her heart 12 years ago. She had been taking prescribed medication and, in addition, had optimized her nutrition with a healthy diet and nutritional supplements. It seemed she was doing all she could possibly do to help her heart. In spite of her committed health program, she was still always tired and very weak.

One day Jodi was amazed to see this patient arrive to the clinic with a spring in her step and a radiant glow to her face. She announced that she had been sleeping so much better in addition to feeling more energy, which was evident to all the staff. She felt better than she had in years. When queried about her impressive improvement, she told everyone it was absolutely due to Salba that she was faithfully adding to her diet on a daily basis.

This Salba convert now is an enthusiastic ambassador of the Salba message. She tells everyone about her amazing recovery. She has also successfully converted all her family member as well as friends into loyal Salba fans as well

Jodi also believes the Salba was the reason for her patient's renewed vitality since nothing else in her program had changed. "Although all the supplements she was taking had helped her heart function, getting the added nutrition from Salba had tipped her over into a new level of wellbeing."

According to Jodi who is a Salba fan herself, "Coming from an understanding of whole foods, we are getting much more nutrition from Salba than we realize. It's not just Salba's high Omega 3 content (which is definitely heart healthy), it's all the other nutrients in that little seed which ultimately will help it grow into a healthy plant. The wisdom of our body knows how to utilize all the nourishment that is packed into those tiny Salba seeds. It truly is Nature's perfect food."

Kat James

Health Educator and Author

If there ever was woman on a mission, it is Kat James, author of the bestselling book, *The Truth About Beauty*. Kat transformed her body and skin beyond recognition after a 12-year eating disorder and liver disorder nearly took her life. She has since, through her book, national health column, PBS special, worldwide talks and Total Transformation® Programs, helped millions to mastermind their own successful "extreme makeovers" using science and strategy, rather than suffering or using dangerous and short-lived extreme measures.

Kat has a list of super foods that she recommends for good health. Salba is on the top of that list because, "Deep, dense nutrition and avoiding blood sugar spikes are the two governing principles of the food aspect of my program. Salba is an unbeatable tool for achieving both objectives. At my Total Transformation® Programs and at home, I incorporate Salba into just about any recipes—from my chocolate-covered Salba nut balls (see recipe chapter) , to my lamb meatloaf (instead of breadcrumbs), to the crust of my low-glycemic cheesecake. If everyone merely tweaked their existing recipes with Salba—which lowers a food's impact on blood sugar—we might have a transformation in physical appearance and transformation in wellbeing."

Kat is always exploring the best nutritional options to enhance a person's life long vitality. For her, Salba is an essential ingredient for vibrant health. "Just like any negative habit shapes us and largely determines what we'll see in the mirror— and how we feel—a decade or more down the road, as well as tomorrow, just making each meal more nourishing and minimizing

its blood sugar impact with the help of Salba, can transform your future, literally! I have many people who've attended my program who—like me—use Salba constantly—all for their own reasons. Some use it in their smoothies for regularity. Many, to help their diabetes, since the research is so compelling, use it to help avoid cravings, and some to thicken their soups and sauces.

For Kat, her vitality and health would not be the same without Salba.

Vitality at Any Age

IT'S JUST COMMON SENSE. The quality of the food we put into our body will determine the quality of its functioning. Whatever dietary program you have chosen in your quest for optimal wellbeing, Salba should certainly be a partner along the way. You can enhance any meal with a whole food source that contains all the building blocks for life: omega 3 fatty acids, minerals, vitamins, antioxidants, fiber and protein. There's no excuse not to use Salba every day. It's not only super nutritious but also super versatile. Whether it takes the starring role in a dish or is incognito as a hidden ingredient, one thing is for sure…. you are on the road to lifelong vitality.

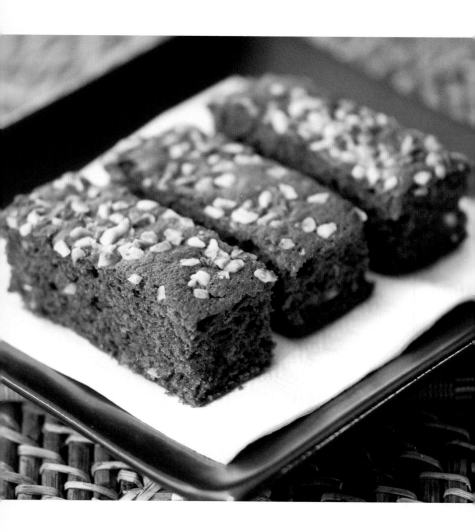

CHAPTER NINE

SALBA
RECIPES

Salba Recipes

Ways to Use Salba

Salba Seeds are amazingly versatile. The easiest way to incorporate Salba into your daily dietary program is to use the whole seeds, either sprinkling them directly on foods or adding the seeds to your recipes.

As you experiment with the many ways Salba can be a part of any dish, you will see the many possibilities of enhancing the nutritional profile of just about any recipe. Just let your creativity free!

Salba is also available already ground for our convenience. However, if you choose to grind Salba yourself you will need to use a coffee grinder. Store any extra ground Salba in the refrigerator.

Use a minimum 2 tbsp of whole or ground Salba daily for optimum nutritional benefits.

USES FOR GROUND SALBA

Gravy thickener, soup, oatmeal, as an extender for hamburgers, in baked goods, etc.

When baking, use 3 parts flour and 1 part ground Salba.

HOW TO MAKE SALBA GEL

Salba gel is another way to use Salba. By soaking the seeds, they become soft and mucilaginous. It is Salba without the crunchiness. The gel texture can then be used to thicken

dishes i.e. soups, stews, gravies, sauces, salad dressings, smoothies, drinks etc. It can also be used as an egg replacement in baking.

In a jar with a tight fitting lid, put 3 cups slightly warm water and 1/2 cup Salba. Cap and shake jar vigorously for 15 seconds. Let stand 1 minute and shake again

Allow to set up for 15 minutes before using. Keep refrigerated. It will keep up to 2 weeks, for later use in recipes.

For example Salba gel can be added to many foods and drinks. Try using half Salba gel and half juice (of any kind). Can also be added to salad dressings, dips, spreads, soups, etc.

The gel can be added to creamy/liquid food items such as jelly, jam, yogurt, mustard, ketchup, salad dressing, barbecue sauce, puddings, yogurt, hot and cold beverages, etc.

The gel doesn't affect flavors, offers nutritional benefits, and cuts calories by decreasing the amount of the food item being extended or displaced.

1/4 cup of Salba gel replaces 1 egg in recipes.

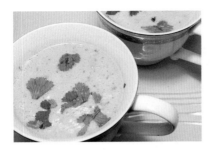

Salba Awesome Avocado Soup

This soup is full of flavor and the avocado makes the soup unbelievably tasty and creamy. This soup is also perfect for a dinner party to surprise your friends.

Makes 2 servings

INGREDIENTS:

* 1 large ripe avocado
* 2 tbsp lemon juice
* 1 tsp olive oil
* 3/4 cup canned corn kernels, drained
* 2 tomatoes, peeled and seeded, chopped
* 1 leek, chopped
* 1 garlic clove, chopped
* 2 cup vegetable broth
* 1/4 cup Salba whole seed, soaked in 3/4 cup of water

DIRECTIONS:

Peel the avocado, remove the nut and mash with a fork, stir in lemon juice and reserve until needed. Heat the olive oil. Add corn, tomatoes, garlic, leek, and garlic. Sauté on low heat for 5-6 minutes until soft. Put half of the vegetables mixture in a food processor or blender, together with the mashed avocado, the Salba gel and the hot vegetable broth. Process until smooth. Transfer the mixture to a clean pot. Add the remaining vegetables. Garnish with corn kernels, red chili or parsley.

Herbed Ricotta Spread

A perfect spread for pita or crackers. Always a party favorite.

INGREDIENTS:

* 1 cup ricotta
* 1/2 cup Salba seeds
* 1/2 tbsp chopped parsley
* 1/2 tbsp chopped cilantro
* 1/2 tbsp chopped rosemary sprigs

DIRECTIONS:

In a bowl, combine the ingredients and mix well, Spread on crackers, crostini, or raw sliced veggies.

Tomato Basil Salad Dressing

INGREDIENTS:

* 2 tomatoes
* 2 tbsp apple cider vinegar
* 1 tbsp Salba Gel
* 2 tbsp Salba Seed Oil
* 1 tbsp dried basil (or 3 tbsp fresh)
* 1 tbsp agave nectar
* Black pepper and sea salt to taste

Makes about 1 1/2 cups.

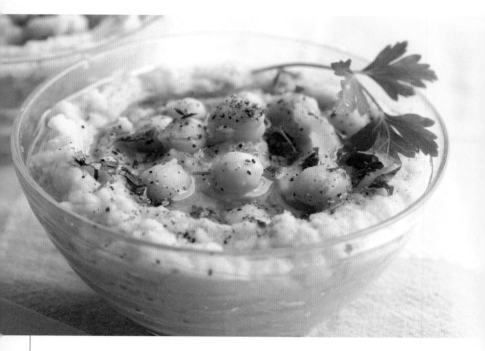

Salba Irish Hummus

Hummus is a chickpea paste that is popular in various local forms throughout the Middle East, but its origins are unknown. In Arabic the word hummus is used to describe the dish or just chickpeas.

Makes 2.5 cups

INGREDIENTS:

* 1 cup chickpeas from a can, drained
* 1/2 lemon, juice
* 1 clove garlic
* 1/4 cup olive oil
* 1/4 cup sunflower oil
* 1-cup fresh parsley (keep some parsley for garnish)
* 1/4 tsp chili powder
* 1/2-cup water
* 1/2 tsp unrefined sea salt
* 2 tbsp Salba whole seed

DIRECTIONS:

Mix all the ingredients with a blender until it is smooth and creamy. Garnish with parsley. Serve with toast, crackers or vegetable sticks.

Salba Bean Salad

Beans are called a 'super food' for good reason. Everyone knows they are an excellent source of protein and fiber, but did you know they are also a good source of thiamin, iron, folate and potassium? Studies note beans are also a great source of antioxidants; the darker bean's color, the more antioxidants they have.

Makes 1 bowl

* 1 1/2 cups frozen shelled edamame (8 oz)
* 1/4 cup olive oil
* 1 teaspoon ground cumin
* 1 (15-oz) can black beans, drained and rinsed
* 1 (15-oz) can black-eyed peas, drained and rinsed
* 1/2 cup chopped red onion
* 2 cups (about 4 stalks) thinly sliced celery
* Zest and juice from 1 lime
* 1/2 cup chopped fresh cilantro
* 2 cloves finely chopped garlic
* 1 1/2 teaspoons salt
* 1/4 teaspoon black pepper
* 4 tbsp Saba whole seed

Heat oil in a small heavy skillet over moderately low heat until hot but not smoking. Add the cumin, stirring, until fragrant, about 30 seconds. Pour into a large heatproof bowl. Add edamame and remaining ingredients to cumin oil and mix well. Let stand 10 minutes for the flavors to blend.

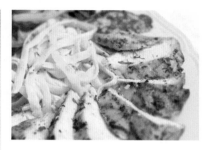

Salba Fettuccini Alfredo with Chicken Piccata
(By Linda Barrett)

This is an Omega-3 rich high protein entrée with the added benefit of being fiber and antioxidant-rich. It's sure to be a hit when you want to serve that 'special' dinner that's also healthy. You can enjoy this dish even if you're a vegetarian. (Chicken substitute could be Morning Star Farms® Veggie Chicken Strips.)

Prepare your favorite Fettuccini Alfredo (or gluten-free pasta) to serve 6 with this recipe. Add 2 cups of 'Salba gel' to the Alfredo Sauce before mixing with fettuccini noodles. For an added antioxidant and fiber boost add 5 tbsp or more chopped basil (Purple Opal basil is exceptional) to the sauce. You may want to prepare the Fettuccini Alfredo in advance and bake at 350° for 30 minutes in a large casserole dish while preparing Chicken Picatta.

INGREDIENTS:

* 1 lb skinless, boneless chicken breast halves
* 2 tbsp unbleached all purpose flour
* 2 tbsp butter (softened)
* ½ salt and pepper (white pepper is exceptionally good in this recipe) to taste
* 4 tbsp Coconut oil

TO PREPARE CHICKEN:

Place chicken in a strong freezer bag and place on a cutting board. Lightly pound chicken to ½ inch thickness. Sprinkle chicken with salt and pepper (white preferably). Dust the chicken in white whole wheat flour or gluten-free flour. Heat a frying pan to medium heat. Add 2 tbsp coconut oil to pan and place chicken breasts into pan. Sauté each side until golden brown, about 10 minutes on each side or to taste. Turn heat off and cover to keep warm.

TO PREPARE SALBA SAUCE:

* 1/2 cup dry white wine
* 1/3-cup fresh lemon juice
* 1/2 cup chicken broth—vegetable broth for veggie chicken
* 1/3 cup drained capers
* 1/3 cup chopped fresh Italian parsley
* 1 1/2 cups Salba gel

DIRECTIONS:

Mix 1 tbsp butter with 2 tbsp all-purpose flour until smooth. Mix wine, lemon juice and broth in a medium saucepan and turn to medium heat.

Bring wine/lemon liquid to a simmer and whisk in the butter/flour mixture. Simmer on a very low boil for about 2 minutes until it thickens. Stir in capers, parsley and remaining 2 tbsp coconut oil. Add 1 1/2cups Salba gel and heat.

Place chicken or veggie chicken strips in a serving dish. Pour Salba sauce over the chicken. Decorate top with lemon and a sprig of Italian parsley. Serve over reduced-calorie fettuccini. Enjoy! Your guests will be convinced you are a gourmet cook...and they will be doubly impressed when they learn its fiber and Omega-3 rich and loaded with age-defying antioxidants.

Salba Baked Swiss Italian Polenta

(By Linda Barrett)

This is a healthy dish that will be sure to bring requests for more. It really tastes too good to be so healthy. Salba is the perfect ingredient to create the balance between Omega-3 and Omega-6, which is high in corn. This nutrient rich recipe is simple to make and well worth the effort.

Polenta must be prepared 2 to 3 hours before (can reduce time by setting in the refrigerator after most of the heat is gone, but don't freeze) or prepare the day before to give Polenta time to set.

Prepare the Salba gel first, to use

in preparing the Polenta. Why not make extra to keep refrigerated to easily add to so many foods to lower calories-per-serving, while adding an Omega-3, antioxidant and fiber boost. Salba gel also aids in digestion to help prevent heartburn.

SALBA GEL: In a jar with a tight fitting lid, put 3 cups slightly warm water and 1/2 cup Salba. Cap and shake jar vigorously for 15 seconds. Let stand 1 minute and shake again. Let stand while cooking Polenta.

With the gel that's left over, try adding a 1 tbsp per pancake to your mix for the best pancakes you ever made, or add 3 tbsp to a glass of orange juice...use your imagination...there's hardly anything you can't add this nutrient/energy boost to, as it doesn't alter flavor.

TO MAKE POLENTA:

* 4 cups pure water
* 1 tsp sea salt
* 1 cup Polenta (coarse cornmeal found in the baking aisle of most supermarkets)
* 1 cup Salba gel
* 4 large garlic cloves (chopped)
* 4 tbsp chopped fresh basil (Purple Opal and Genovese or any basil available)
* 4 tbsp chopped Italian Parsley

1. In a large, thick-bottomed saucepan, put water and sea salt. Bring to a boil. Pour Polenta into water

while rapidly whisking. Bring back to a boil while mixing. Turn heat down to lowest setting and cover with a splatter screen. Continue cooking for 20 minutes, stirring with a wooden spoon often. (Quicker cooking cornmeal may be used instead of Polenta meal, but the authentic taste of Polenta is definitely worth the extra effort. Follow the directions on the box to cook quick cornmeal, if desired, using recipe for 4 cups water and continue.)

2. Add the Salba gel, basil and Italian parsley and mix very well.

3. Pour Polenta into a lightly oiled 8 or 9-inch square glass baking pan. Let cool uncovered 1 hr. Let cool completely 1 or 2 hrs to set or place in the refrigerator overnight.

TO MAKE TOMATO SAUCE:

* 2 tbsp olive oil
* 1 medium onion, diced fine
* 1 small red bell pepper, diced fine
* 2 cloves garlic, crushed
* 10 anise seeds, crushed
* Dash of nutmeg
* 6 medium tomatoes (28 oz), diced (or 2-14oz cans diced tomatoes)
* 2 tbsp tomato puree
* 1 tbsp maple syrup
* 1 cup Salba gel
* Salt and pepper to taste
* 3 oz Gruyère cheese, finely shredded

1. Heat a large pot on medium high heat. Add olive oil and onion. Sauté 1 minute and add bell pepper and crushed garlic. Sauté until onions are light brown.

2. Add anise and nutmeg and sauté for 1 more minute. Add diced tomatoes, tomato puree and maple syrup. Bring to a simmer and turn to low. Simmer for up to 1 hr covered with a spatter screen, until sauce is a good, thick consistency. Add the Salba gel and mix well.

3. While sauce is simmering, cut polenta into cubes about ¾ inch thick, whatever square or rectangle shape you desire.

4. Arrange in a lightly oiled casserole dish. Spoon tomato sauce over 1st layer and sprinkle ½ of the shredded cheese over the sauce. Repeat another layer with Polenta, tomato sauce and Gruyère cheese.

5. Bake in a preheated 400° oven for 25 to 30 minutes until golden brown and cheese is nicely melted.

Serve Salba Polenta over pasta with your favorite red sauce with 11/2 cups Salba added to it, or double the recipe for the Polenta sauce and use it with your favorite pasta. Spoon the Polenta on top of the pasta and sauce when serving. This super low-calorie meal will be sure to please the heartiest of appetites. Enjoy this authentic Italian dish with the influence of California's version of health.

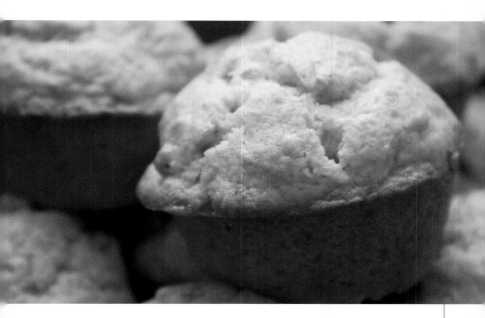

Salba Banana Coconut Muffins

This is a scrumptious gluten-free and sugar- free muffin recipe.

Makes 6 muffins

INGREDIENTS:

* 2 Tbsp coconut oil
* 3 room-temperature eggs
* 1/3 cup mashed banana (1 small ripe banana)
* 1 tsp. alcohol-free vanilla flavor or vanilla extract
* 1/4 tsp salt
* 1/4 cup coconut flour
* 2 tbsp Salba Seeds
* 1/4 tsp baking powder
* 1/2 tsp ground cinnamon
* 1 tbsp shredded coconut
* 2 tbsp raisins, cranberries or blueberries (optional)

DIRECTIONS:

Preheat oven to 400ºF. Mix together oil, eggs, banana, vanilla, and salt.

Add coconut flour, Salba, baking powder, cinnamon, and shredded coconut, and whisk together until smooth.

Fold in raisins. Other options include dried cranberries, blueberries, walnuts, cashews or cacao nibs.

Pour into muffin cups greased with coconut oil.

Bake 15 minutes or until toothpick inserted in center of muffins comes out clean. Cool on wire rack.

Homemade Salba Granola

Makes about 12 cups of super fresh low-cost cereal.

INGREDIENTS:

* 4 cups peanuts
* 2 cups sunflower seeds
* 4 cups rolled oats
* 1 cup whole Salba seeds
* 2 cups wheat germ
* 1/4 cup oil
* 1/4 cup maple syrup

DIRECTIONS:

Grind up the nuts and seeds in a food processor for 2 pulses. If you don't have a food processor, leave everything whole. Combine everything and place on an oven tray and bake for one hour at 350°F, stirring the granola every 20 minutes.

Variations: Use other kinds of nuts such as cashews, walnuts, almonds or hazelnuts.

Salba Pudding (Raw Food and Gluten-Free)

INGREDIENTS:

* 2 tbsp Salba seeds
* 1 cup Nut Milk (Recipe to Follow)
* Strawberries, banana, kiwi, blueberry or mango to garnish

DIRECTIONS:

In a bowl stir the Salba seeds into the Nut Milk and whisk to break up any clumps. Allow the mixture to set for 30 min - 1 hr, whisking occasionally. Garnish each serving with your choice of fruit.

Nut Milk

INGREDIENTS:

* 1 cup raw almonds or cashews, soaked overnight, drained and rinsed
* 4 cups water
* 1 ea vanilla bean or 1 tsp vanilla extract
* 4 ea dates or sweetener of choice (Honey, Agave, Stevia)
* 1/4 - 1/2 tsp celtic sea salt

DIRECTIONS:

Blend the nuts and water on high speed. Strain the liquid through a Nut Milk bag, cheesecloth or fine mesh strainer. Reserve the 'nut meat' for another use and place the Nut Milk back into the blender. Add the remaining ingredients and blend until smooth. Adjust seasonings to taste.

Salba Fudge Nut Brownies

Salba makes yummy treats that taste moist and decadent. Set out a plateful and poof -- they'll be gone!

INGREDIENTS:

* 1 lb semi-sweet chocolate morsels
* 1 1/4 cup all purpose flour
* 1 cup butter
* 4 medium eggs
* 1 cup hazelnuts

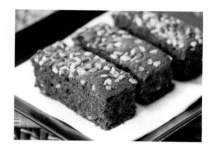

* 5 tbsp Salba (Use Ground Salba or grind Salba seeds in a coffee grinder)
* 1/4 tsp salt
* 1 cup sugar
* 2 tsp vanilla extract

DIRECTIONS:

In a heavy saucepan, melt chocolate chips and butter. Add sugar, Salba and salt, and stir until dissolved. Cool for 10 minutes. Stir in beaten eggs, vanilla extract, flour and nuts.

Pour into a greased, 15 x 10 x 1 baking pan. Bake at 350° for 25-30 minutes, or until a tooth pick inserted near the corners comes out with moist crumbs. Let sit to cool.

Makes 2 1/2 dozen brownies.

Kat's Deep Chocolate Salba Nut Balls
(Created by Kat James)

These nut butter and Saba balls which I make as a group at my Total Transformation® programs are the perfect anytime, on-the-run, never- skip-a-meal, never-a-craving, decadent snack choice that will never spike your blood sugar if the sweetener is smart. Great straight out of the freezer and to keep the kids happy. Perfect in place of expensive, sweetened energy bars, and the perfect frozen candy bar upgrade. Even makes a great breakfast.

Makes 16-20 balls.

Basic Nut Ball Mixture

INGREDIENTS:

* 1 16-oz. jar of nut butter, such as almond, peanut, walnut, or a mixture
* 1/2 cup unsweetened, quality whey protein powder (vanilla whey powder adds a nice flavor)
* 1/3 cup liquefied virgin coconut oil, (to liquefy, just run hot water over the jar until oil is clear)
* 1/3-1/2 cup ground Salba (The more Salba, the more nourishing these balls are.)
* Smart sweetener to taste, like de-bittered stevia or xylitol
* 1/2-1 tsp sea salt, depending on how much salt is in the nut butter you use (the saltiness plays well against the sweetness of the chocolate)

Optional: unsweetened natural flavorings or extracts, such as walnut, almond, coconut, cherry (available from Frontier), or spices like cinnamon or nutmeg.

DIRECTIONS:

Mix together the above ingredients (and any additional optional filling ingredients below) in a large bowl (adjusting sweetness and flavorings to taste). Freeze for an hour or so to achieve workable texture to facilitate palm-rolling into walnut-sized balls. Freeze balls again before rolling in coatings below.

Optional Filling or Coating Ingredients

The following can either be blended into the ball mixture, or rolled on the surface of the frozen balls, before or after dipping in the melted chocolate mixture (I recommend re-freezing balls after rolling so they can be dipped into the melted chocolate without falling apart):

* Unsweetened shredded coconut
* Roasted crushed nuts or sesame seeds
* Dried goji berries

Melted Chocolate Coating

INGREDIENTS:

* 6 oz. unsweetened chocolate
* 2 tbsp organic butter or virgin coconut oil
* Smart sweetener to taste. I often use a few drops of vanilla stevia liquid for this.

DIRECTIONS:

Place the above ingredients together in a double boiler or a metal bowl over simmering water, stirring occasionally until melted. Dip the frozen balls into the melted chocolate mixture covering them completely, then place a half an inch apart on a cookie sheet or in a brownie pan in the freezer until set.

Salba Tahini Banana Dream Drink

This drink is fast to make and contains lots of calcium from the Salba and tahini (sesame seed butter).

Makes 2 drinks

INGREDIENTS:

* 2 tbsp tahini
* 1 banana
* 1 cup rice milk
* 2 tbsp Salba

DIRECTIONS:

Blend the banana, tahini, Salba and milk together.

Basic Electrolyte Sport Drink

* 3 parts of your favorite unsweetened fruit juice (use fresh, not pasteurized, juice to make juice 100% raw)
* 1 part water
* 1 tbsp Salba seeds or gel
* Sea salt to taste

DIRECTIONS:

Combine all ingredients in a water bottle or cup. Stir thoroughly.

Lemon-Lime Gel (Raw food and gluten free)

INGREDIENTS:

* 1/2 cup agave nectar
* 1 tbsp lime zest
* 1 tsp lemon zest
* 1 tbsp Salba seeds or gel
* 1/2 tsp dulse (seaweed)
* Sea salt to taste

DIRECTIONS:

In a blender, combine all ingredients; process until blend reaches a gel-like consistency. This gel will keep for up to 3 days in the refrigerator, but it is best when consumed fresh.

Direct Fuel Bites

INGREDIENTS:

* 5 dates
* 2 tbsp coconut oil
* 2 tsp lemon zest
* 1 tsp lemon juice
* 1 tbsp Salba seeds or gel
* Sea salt to taste

DIRECTIONS:

In a food processor, combine all ingredients; process until smooth. Form mixture into a 1/2 inch-think rectangle. Cut into bite-size pieces. Individually wrap in cellophane and store in the refrigerator or freezer.

Will keep well in freezer for up to 3 months, and for up to 2 weeks in the refrigerator.

Fast Fuel Gels

These gels can be stored in small plastic zip-up bags and taken with you for a long workout or race. However, they are easier to handle and consume when put into a flask, which can be bought at most sunning-supply stores.

Chocolate Blueberry Energy Bars

INGREDIENTS:

* 1 cup fresh or soaked dried dates
* 1/4 cup almonds
* 1/4 cup blueberries (fresh or frozen)
* 1/4 cup roasted carob powder
* 1/4 cup Salba seeds or gel
* 1/4 cup hemp protein
* 1/4 cup unhulled sesame seeds
* 1 tsp fresh lemon juice
* 1/2 tsp lemon zest
* Sea salt to taste

DIRECTIONS:

Knead berries into mixture by hand.

In a food processor, process all ingredients until desired texture is reached. If you want a crunchy texture, blend less.

Remove mixture from processor and put on a clean surface. There are two ways to shape the bars. You could roll the mixture into several balls or shape it into bars.

To shape as bars, flatten mixture on the clean surface with your hands. Place plastic wrap over top; with a rolling pin, roll mixture to desired bar thickness. Cut into bars or form into a brick, cut as though slicing bread.

Recovery Pudding

This pudding tastes especially good when cold, just after a hot summer workout.

* 2 bananas
* 1 cup blueberries
* 1/2 cups soaked almonds
* 1/4 cup Salba seeds
* 1/4 cup hemp protein
* 1/4 cup roasted carob powder
* 1 tsp lemon juice
* 1/4 tsp sea salt

DIRECTIONS:

In a food processor, combine all ingredients; process until smooth.

This pudding will keep for up to 3 days in the refrigerator, but it is best when eaten fresh.

SALBA
EXPERIENCES

Much Improved Digestion

After two weeks of taking the Salba my husband asked me what happened to my stomach. Before the Salba, no matter what I ate or took I had indigestion, constipation, cold hands and feet, low energy, as well as fluctuation in my blood pressure. I have personally found that the best results for me included taking 1 tbsp of gel-forming Salba seed in the morning followed by a cup of hot lemon water, and 1 tbsp of gel-forming Salba seed before bedtime. In addition I add ground Salba to soups, salads and baking. Have never felt better, thanks Salba.

S. Ch.

Great Improvement in Energy, Hunger and Weight Loss

After taking Salba for only a week or two, I noticed my energy level had risen. I also lost four excess pounds very quickly. I used to snack a lot, but after starting Salba, I would go to the fridge, look in, and decide; I really wasn't hungry. Salba has also lowered my blood glucose readings. My levels would always spike after meals, and with Salba they remain lower and more constant. I take it first thing in the morning so that I have plenty of time to use up the extra energy before bedtime. My favorite use is in sugar-free yogurt at breakfast, but I also put it in soup, cereal, and salads. I have experienced a noticeable improvement in vim, vigor, and mood.

Barbara

Stabilized Blood Sugar Levels

I am a type 2 diabetic, after taking Salba for two weeks, my blood sugar has stabilized. I have lost 7 pounds, and have more energy! I also notice my blood pressure has gone down due to more exercise and Salba. Also with the high fiber content of Salba, my bowel movements have become regular. Salba can be used with anything, and there is no after taste.

M. Robinson

A Versatile Food

It is so versatile, and can be used in so many ways. I sprinkled it in its whole seed version on salads, coleslaw, cottage cheese, yogurt, and oatmeal. In addition, I included it when baking oatmeal, corn bread, and bran muffins. It was so delicious in smoothies. I've been using flaxseed for years, but Salba seems to add so much more!

C. Harmon

More Energy and Less Appetite

This product came at an opportune time. I have just been diagnosed as borderline diabetic. When I started taking this, it truly made a difference. I received more energy to do the things I needed to do. It also curbed my appetite so that I didn't crave certain foods. Overall I feel a lot better.

S. Gideon

Improved Skin and Energy Levels

I used this product for 2 weeks and noticed the ton of energy Salba has given me! My skin has cleared up, thanks to all the Omegas. These little seeds are so easy to incorporate into dishes and they have absolutely no taste. When ground up, my children cannot detect them!

S. White

Great Nutrition for the Family

Salba arrived at my door like a miracle. My husband just had a stent placed in his heart valve and I was looking to up my fiber. I am able to grind it and put it in my husband and children's foods undetected.

F. Freedman

No More Afternoon Slump

After using Salba for 10 days, the main benefit I noticed was increased stamina throughout the day. No more afternoon slump.

G. Moran

Great Nutritional Value

I love this product because of the wonderful nutritional values it contains. We get more calcium, magnesium, antioxidants and fish oils in our diet and this provides it all in one.

D. Quale

Indigestion Gone

For months I was having stomach difficulties. Anytime I would lie down, I would suffer from severe indigestion and was unable to keep down any food. Needless to say, I slept sitting up all the time. I was prescribed several different types of medication and nothing worked... after taking the product (Salba) for only 1 day I was sleeping in my bed. After two weeks of taking the Salba I decided to take a break from it to find out if it was truly the Salba that was making me feel better. The next day I was back sleeping in my chair again. In addition to sleep, I have lost inches and regained energy. Thanks Salba.

M. Woodstock

Increased Energy, Glowing Skin

As a nutritional biochemist, I am always looking for new whole foods that my clients can incorporate into their diet. (With Salba) Many people found they received increased energy, less blood sugar swings, and better moods. There was even a marked glow to the women's skin - wrinkles were also less visible as (Salba's) EFA's plumped up their skin! I heartily recommend it to all my clients now. It seems to help with low level depression (especially the Seasonal Affective Disorder so many Northerners get this time of year), food cravings and increase sports stamina.

M. Keener

Better Shape Than 15-20 Years Ago

Today, my family started our annual pre-spring cleaning of our back yard... to my surprise I found myself to be physically in better shape now than perhaps 15-20 years ago and perform the heavy labor to prepare the grounds as required. It's amazing when you are in the regime of taking Salba you don't feel super power wellness until you put your body to task. After having taken medication for nearly 20 years, with which I never reached my current plateau readings of 123/72 with a pulse rate of 65, I'm happy to inform you that I have reached my personal goal that I have longed to reach.

M. Guerrero

Great for Baking

I'm lovin' this stuff! Easy to grind, easy to store and wonderful to bake with! So far the waffles are excellent, cookies are delightful, sauces and gravies are easily thickened and oh the broth turned out perfectly for homemade chicken and noodles! I believe I've only just begun to experiment... I typically do a lot more in the kitchen as the weather cools off and winter months keep us nestled in. Need I say more? Keep it well stocked!

C. Banta

Renewed Energy for Sports

My name is Gene and I am a relatively new user of Salba. I am 25 years old and am very active. I work out nearly every day, weight train and rollerblade as much as my schedule allows and it's very hard for me to find the energy to get up and go lots of the time. However, since I've started having a Salba shake in the mornings each day I've noticed vast amounts of energy at times in the day when before I'd feel drained. I can honestly say this is one of the best products I've tried. Not only does it work, but it's versatile as well. It can be added into nearly anything without affecting flavor or cook time. I will definitely continue to use this product.

G. Wesselius

Solved Chronic Digestive Problems

I bought three bags of Salba and I am now totally committed to this product. My digestive problems have seemed to worsen in recent years. After all the products the naturopathic people have had me try, it is hard to believe that this little grain does the trick. And, it can be carried around easily when one travels. I LOVE IT. Have been talking it up to anyone who will listen. I have my husband on it as well. I am very grateful for the recommendation.

J. Samson

Used as Part of Health Care Program

I have been an integrative medical professional for over 20 years. When I first heard about Salba, I thought it was one of the many nutritional products on the market with unrealistic claims and little or no research or results

to back them up. Surprisingly, after further review and personal use of this amazing product, I have found it truly is the Most Powerful Super grain. Salba is incredible; its health properties are exemplary. I am excited about the opportunity to integrate Salba into my health care protocols. It is truly remarkable that something with this much nutritional value tastes fantastic, with no odor or aftertaste and can be easily assimilated into virtually any food regime.

Dr. Derrick DeSilva, Jr., M.D.

Getting Real Nutrition

I used to take a lot of supplements... vitamin C, potassium, iron, calcium... omega-3s. And now, I'm just simply adding 2 tablespoons of Salba to my morning cereal, oatmeal, or yogurt.

Joanne

Health Recovery for 12 Year Old Dog

Lolli, my 12 year Yorkie was diagnosed with diabetes and Cushing's disease in 12/06. While working at the Center for Integrative Health I overheard the health coach as well as the physicians talk about Salba and how great this product is not only for healthy people but especially for diabetics because it is supposed to keep blood sugars even throughout the day due to its fiber content. I began to think - why not? If Salba is good for people, why not my dog. I began to put 1/2 teaspoon of Salba on Lolli's food twice daily beginning the last week in February 2008. Below are Lolli's blood work ups - January 3, 2008 (with out Salba) and March 20, 2008 with Salba:

January 3, 2008 (Without Salba)
Glucose at 354
(ref range 70-138mg/dl)
Lipase 1196
(ref range 77-695 U/L)
Amylase 1564
(ref range 290-1125 U/L)

Triglycerides 704
(ref range 59-291 mg/dl)
Cholesterol 496
(ref range 92-324 mg/dl)

March 20, 2008 (With Salba)

Glucose 284	70 point drop
Lipase 660	536 point drop
Amylase 768	796 point drop
Triglycerides 602	102 point drop
Cholesterol 437	59 point drop

After receiving the above results, I was one happy puppy!

P.S. Lolli loves Salba - she has no problem eating after I sprinkle Salba on her meals and she is one <u>picky</u> eater.

N. Catinella

FREQUENTLY ASKED QUESTIONS

What is Salba?

Salba is a 100 percent natural whole grain packed with more energizing nutrition than any other grain, even flax. In fact, after more than a decade of testing, no single food is known to match Salba's nutritive power. Salba is rich in omega-3 fatty acids, beneficial fiber, calcium, magnesium, iron, Vitamin C, potassium, vegetable proteins plus vital age-fighting antioxidants. Studies suggest Salba's unique nutritional make-up can help boost your energy, improve your heart health, enhance your memory and mood, strengthen your joint mobility and bone health, promote balanced blood sugar and a healthy weight, fortify your immune system, support easy digestion and even help defend against aging and degenerative disease.

Where does Salba come from?

Salba grows in South America. This grain, in one form or another, has been around for more than 500 years. In ancient times the Aztecs valued it more highly than gold, and for good reason. Salba is chock full of body-fueling fatty acids, vitamins, minerals and antioxidants. What's more, nutrition scientists realized by harvesting only specific grains (the white ones) they can enhance the nutrient density of this super-grain even further.

Where is Salba grown?

Today Salba is grown under controlled conditions in some of the most nutrient-rich soil in the world, in the pristine land surrounding the Amazon Basin in Peru. Because the soil's natural nutrient stores have never been depleted, Salba is packed with more naturally occurring beneficial vitamins and minerals than many fruits, vegetables and dairy products farmed elsewhere. Salba is 100 percent natural.

Who should use Salba?

Everyone. Because of Salba's nutritional density, this super-grain is beneficial to people of every age. For instance:

* **Salba can help provide the key nutrients children and adolescents need to develop into strong, healthy adults.**

* **It can replenish essential antioxidants and minerals in athletes, which are leeched away by their high level of physical activity.**

* Salba's rich calcium and iron content make it excellent for women in their childbearing years and beyond menopause.

* Its high fiber content makes Salba a great help to those watching their weight. Salba helps alleviate feelings of hunger while helping cleanse the colon and bowels for more effective digestion.

* Salba's superior ratio of omega-3 fatty acids, fiber, antioxidants and minerals make it perfect for anyone concerned about fighting the process of aging. Studies show these nutrients help reduce fatigue, strengthen your heart muscle, improve blood circulation and flow, support healthy blood sugar levels, promote agile joints, improve digestion even enhance mental clarity and memory.

How do I take Salba?

To maintain Salba's exceptional nutritional profile it's not encapsulated or manufactured into any kind of tablet or gel cap. Instead, you'll enjoy Salba just as nature intended, as a whole grain. You can sprinkle Salba on cereal in the morning or mix it with yogurt, smoothies or salads. You can also use Salba to cook with, putting it in burgers, soups, casseroles, pastas or anything else. And it's great for baking too; you can replace 10-25 percent of flour in any recipe with ground Salba. Put Salba in cookies or cakes and transform a favorite tasty treat into one that's packed with nutrition. Try it; you'll enjoy this kid (and adult) favorite.

How much Salba should I eat?

The suggested serving size is 1 to 2 tablespoons of ground Salba per day, however, up to 5 tablespoons can be consumed daily without negative effects.

Salba is a source of insoluble fiber, which helps to prevent constipation. Drink plenty of fluids and be physically active when increasing fiber intake.

How do I use Salba Oil?

Simply use this oil on foods you eat or to replace oil in salad dressings. Mix it in with yogurt or dips, add it to batters before baking - add to pancake batter, breads, muffins, cakes, cookies, bars, etc. You also can add to meatballs, hamburgers, etc.

What does Salba taste like?

Unlike flaxseed's bitter taste, Salba has no discernable taste. In fact, it tends to take on the flavor of whatever foods or condiments you mix it with so Salba's great with anything from salads to desserts.

Is Salba safe?

Yes. Salba is pure nutrition and 100 percent side-effect free. This natural whole food has gone through more than 15 years of clinical testing and study to prove its safety and nutritional benefits. Salba is the only functional food that is the subject of a medical patent for the ongoing research in the field of diabetic management.

I'm allergic to wheat. Is Salba safe for me?

Absolutely, yes. Salba is 100 percent gluten-free and safe for Celiacs or those with wheat allergies and gluten intolerances.

SALBA VS. CHIA
THE IMPORTANT DIFFERENCES THAT EVERYONE SHOULD KNOW

What is "Chia"?

"Chia" is Latin slang for "oil seed" and describes over five species of "Salvia" plants and refers to all of the 180+ botanical varieties of the one Salvia species: *Salvia hispanica*.[1] Each specie and variety has a different genetic makeup and nutritional component with greater variances by crop location[2], water[3], quality of soil, and other environmental factors. Common "chia" lacks described molecular markers for the species.[4] "Chia" is mostly black or striped with wild and domesticated crops.

What is Salba?

Salba is one specific variety of *Salvia hispanica*. It has two botanical registrations as separate and distinct seed varieties from all other "chia" varieties and is the only food that is the subject of a U.S. medical patent. Salba is the "next generation" of *Salvia hispanica*. By complying with a strict genetic ID program it allows Salba's incredible nutritional components to remain intact: crop after crop.

Location is Everything

The nutritional composition of "chia" is affected by the crop location.[5] Salba is only grown in Peru's pristine Amazon Basin. "Chia" on the market today (both animal and human grade) is mostly grown in Mexico where GMO farming, extensive pesticide/herbicide use and substandard employee practices are common. Mexican "Chia" has greater genetic diversity than other crop locations,[6] making it genetically and morphologically inconsistent.[4] Common "Chia" grown in Mexico lacks described molecular markers for the species. [7]

Facts not Fiction: Medical Research

Salba is the only registered variety of *Salvia hispanica* with intensive human clinical examination and medically published nutrient and health claims. In acute and long-term clinical studies conducted on individuals with Type 2 Diabetes, Salba reduced: (i) after-meal blood glucose and plasma insulin levels (improving insulin sensitivity); (ii) blood pressure; and (iii) risk factors of heart disease such as body inflammation (C-reactive protein (CRP) and coagulation factors (aspirin-like effect).[7] Salba's the first and only grain ever studied to have shown these results. "Chia" seeds are nutritionally inconsistent, have not adhered to Salba's genetic ID program and have not been clinically examined. There is no proof to substantiate that Salba's nutritional fact based evidence can apply in any manner to any other "Chia" seed.

1 USDA United States Department of Agriculture, Natural Resources Conservation Service, Classification, Classification for Kingdom Plantae Down to Genus Salvia L. http://plants.usda.gov.

2 Fatty acid composition, protein, and oil content of "Chia" (*Salvia hispanica L.*) grown in Peru, Columbia, and Argentina, Ayerza (h) & Coates, Southwest Center for Natural Products Research & Commercialization, Office of Arid Land Studies, The University of Arizona, July 31, 2001; and, Composition of chia (*Salvia hispanica*) grown in six tropical and subtropical ecosystems of South America, Ayerza and Coates, Office of Arid Land Studies, The University of Arizona, Trop. Sci., 2004, 44, 131-135.

3 Effect of late salinization of "Chia" (*Salvia hispanica*), stock (Matthiola tricuspidata) and evening primrose (Oenothera biennis) on their oil content and quality, by Bruria Heuer, Zohara Yaniv, and Israela Ravina, March 2002.

4 Genetics of Qualitative Traits in Domesticated Chia (*Salvia hispanica L.*) by J.P. Cahill, and M.C. Provance, Department of Botany and Plant Sciences, Univerity of California, *The Journal of Heredity*, 2002, 93 (1), 52-55.

5 USDA United States department of Agriculture, Seeds, chia seeds, dried, http://www.nal.usda.gov.

6 Genetic diversity among varieties of chia (*Salvia hispanica L.*) by Joseph Cahill, University of California, 2004.

7 Supplementation of Conventional Therapy With the Novel Grain Salba (*Salvia hispanica L.*) Improves Major and Emerging Cardiovascular Risk Factors in Type 2 Diabetes. Vladimir Vuksan et al. *Diabetes Care*, 2007, 30 (11), 2804-2810.

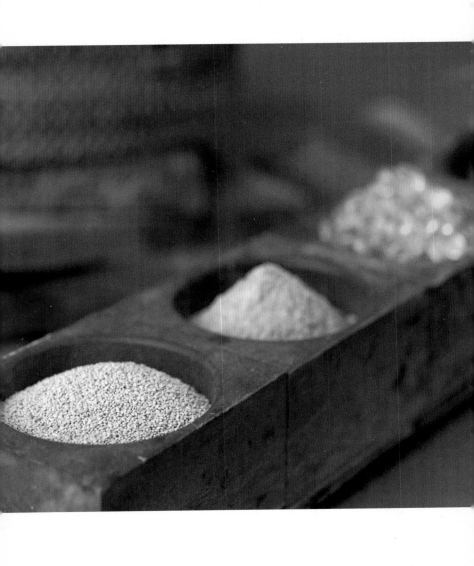

SALBA vs. COMMON CHIA

There are many clear distinctions between common chia seeds and Salba.
Here's a look at a few of the most prominent differences.

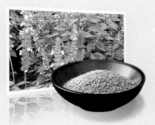

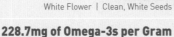

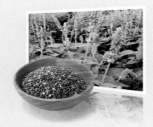

SALBA	CHIA
White Flower | Clean, White Seeds	Bluish-Purple Flower | Dark Seeds
228.7mg of Omega-3s per Gram	**175.5mg of Omega-3s per Gram***
212.0mg of Protein per Gram	**156.2mg of Protein per Gram***
Standardized & Nutritionally Consistent	Inconsistent Nutrient Composition
Grown with Non-GMO Selective Breeding	Typically Grown to Maximize Volume
Evidence-Based: Clinically Researched by Independent Sources	Has Not Undergone Human Clinical Studies
Grown in Peru and Can Be Traced to its Roots	Grown Throughout Central America in Varying Conditions
135 Day Crop Lifecycle; Full Nutrient Maturity	Often Harvested Early to Increase Profitability

*Based on USDA nutritional data.